Praise for *CALORIE QUEENS*

"There is no such thing as coincidence. It was providence that brought Diane and Jackie Scott into our lives after David had a TIA (transient ischemic attack). Their nurturing care and careful planning of our meals blessed us. We continue to benefit from the nutritional balance they have given us through Eucalorics."

—Jackie and David Bondurant

"What an easy read; full of real-life humor and experience. It was a breath of fresh air after years of being bombarded with gimmicky diets! Following a plan that encourages small steps over time is not only a good eating strategy, it's a good life plan for all aspects of living."

—Mary Dodds, owner, North Aire Market

"I have been off and on diets for years and have a bad tendency to use food to deal with stress. As a physician I know what I am supposed to do. When I heard about Eucalorics, it made so much sense and I was glad to have a realistic calorie goal to shoot for instead of unrealistic diets of 700 to 1,000 calories. I already exercised but needed to pay more attention to what I ate. The food is great and the structure of the program is what I needed to get on the right track. My clothes fit better, my exercise endurance is better, and my blood work (cholesterol, triglycerides, etc.) improved during the 12 weeks on the program."

—Melinda G. Rowe, MD,
Eucalorics Healthy Lifestyle Program participant

"This multifaceted program helps you improve not only your weight, but also your health by teaching you to make permanent changes in your eating and exercise habits. It's not designed for quick, easy weight loss; it's designed to help you find a balance between food and exercise that you can live with."
—Pamela Treas, office manager, Eucalorics Healthy Lifestyle Program

Calorie Queens

Living Thin in a Fat World

Jackie Scott and Diane Scott Kellum
with Brett A. Scott, MD

CENTER
STREET

NEW YORK BOSTON NASHVILLE

Center Street

Time Warner Book Group
1271 Avenue of the Americas, New York, NY 10020
Visit our Web site at www.twbookmark.com

The Center Street name and logo are registered trademarks of the Time Warner Book Group.

Printed in the United States of America

First edition: November 2005
10 9 8 7 6 5 4 3 2 1

Library of Congress Cataloging-in-Publication Data
King-Scott, Jackie.
       Calorie queens : living thin in a fat world / Jackie Scott and Diane Scott Kellum with Brett A. Scott.— 1st ed.
          p.   cm.
       Includes bibliographical references and index.
       ISBN 1-931722-59-5
    1. Reducing diets.   I. Scott Kellum, Diane. II. Scott, Brett A. III. Title.

RM222.2.K5426 2005
613.2'5—dc22

                                                                     2005015218

Acknowledgments

This book would not exist without the help of many people, and we're pleased to have the chance to thank some of them. The First United Methodist Church of Lexington, Kentucky, allowed us to use their commercial kitchen, and the participants in the Temple Reconstruction Project ate chef surprise night after night as we developed and perfected the recipes that appear in *Calorie Queens*.

Thanks to Jackie and David Bondurant for love and support, and to John Andrews for true friendship, unending patience.

Stephanie Peterson and Host Communications helped make a work in progress a finished product; Beth White and Joseph Beth Booksellers helped put that product in the right place at the right time. Special thanks to Jennifer Crusie for her excellent taste and timing, and to Christina Hogrebe and Margaret Ruley at the Jane Rotrosen Agency in New York for searching until they found us. Finally, thanks to Christina Boys and Center Street for giving us a chance to become calorie queens.

Contents

Introduction

If you pick up most dictionaries and turn to the word "diet," the first definition doesn't mention weight at all. A diet is supposed to be what a person or animal usually eats and drinks; our daily fare. In today's overweight society, however, most of us are either on a diet or planning to be on a diet, and the word has become synonymous with the unpleasant, unsuccessful, and unending pursuit of weight loss. How did we get so far away from the basic concept of daily fare?

The modern diet era began in 1961, when Dr. Herman Taller published *Calories Don't Count*. There's no evidence that his message descended from a mountain etched on a stone tablet, but over the last few decades this simple phrase has somehow become a fundamental "diet truth" that has supplied the foundation for an assortment of low-carbohydrate-based diet plans. As the steady stream of popular books echoed the calories-don't-count mantra, counting calories became old-fashioned. It was relegated to the realm of outdated and unnecessarily complex practices.

I personally don't find counting to be that difficult a process. Somewhat more involved than learning colors or knowing that a pig says, "Oink," but still pretty fundamental stuff. Everyone knows how to count, right? We can count fingers and toes and money. But ask someone to count calories, and they're suddenly counting-challenged. Suggest that someone keep track of the calories they consume, and suddenly counting becomes an unbearably intricate task. It's especially puzzling because calories are the only thing people find hard to count.

Count fat grams? *Okay. I'll just sit here on the sofa eating fat-free jelly beans and practice for the Couch Potato Olympics.*

Count carbohydrates? *No problem. I'll just snack on these pork rinds until my 24-ounce sirloin arrives.*

Count calories? *Oh dear, I don't think I could possibly manage to do that. Much too complicated.*

Shortly after we drop-kicked calorie counting, Dr. Irwin Stillman's *The Doctor's Quick Weight Loss Book* appeared on the best-seller list. Everybody really liked that title, and "quick weight loss" was carefully chiseled below "calories don't count" on the stone tablet of dieting rules.

If you need to lose ten pounds, *quick* weight loss is possible. If, however, you're in the 31 percent of the population that is classified as obese,[1] you need to lose at least thirty pounds to be a normal weight; for the nearly 5 percent of the population that is morbidly obese,[2] it requires a weight loss of more than one hundred pounds. For most of us, *quick* weight loss is no longer physically possible, but no one wants to admit it.

We've all purchased, perused, and followed an amazing variety of diets that ridiculed counting calories and promised quick weight loss. But while we've been faithfully following the rules of these diet regimes, we've been getting heavier and heavier. Isn't it time to change the rules? Isn't it time for a different approach?

Calorie Queens is a book about losing weight, but it's not a book about dieting. It's a book about eating. Specifically, learning to eat correctly. Every day. Day after day. Forever. It's a book that describes how to make your *diet* your *daily fare* by applying the theories of *Eucalorics* to your life.

What's Eucalorics? The prefix *eu-* means "normal," so a *eucaloric* diet is a *normal-calorie diet*. It is a diet designed to achieve and maintain a healthy weight by consistently consuming the number of calories that support that weight.

If you follow a diet that doesn't provide a sufficient quantity of high-quality food, you'll never stay on it long enough to lose any significant amount of weight. If you follow a diet that says you can never eat at fast-food places and fancy restaurants or have candy, cookies, and chips, you may lose weight, but you have very little chance of keeping the weight off. This is a book about learning to live thin in a fat world so you can lose weight *and not find it again*.

Calorie Queens doesn't start with the words "Once upon a time . . ." but when you read our story, you might think it should. In June of 2000, my daughter, Diane, and I never dreamed we were going to lose three hundred pounds and write a book about a new approach to losing weight. Or that we'd be designing menus and preparing meals for a commercial weight management program being developed in conjunction with a local hospital.

There's a lyric from a wonderful song in Stephen Sondheim's *Merrily We Roll Along* that asks, "How did you get to be here?" When Diane and I talk to people about our personal fairy story, that's what they want to know. How did we get from morbid obesity to our present healthy weights? What changes did we make in our lives? And will our approach to permanent weight loss work for them?

We're hoping that *Calorie Queens* will help you understand how we got to be here, and will help you get here too, so we can all live *happier and healthier ever after*.

Part One

Eucalorics

CHAPTER I

Realistic Expectations

Losing weight is the modern-day quest. The search for the famed city of El Dorado, the fountain of youth, the impossible dream. Most of us have experienced many diet failures, and each failure makes it harder and harder to believe that any long-term solution exists. But we haven't given up hope. We're still looking.

When we're looking for a solution to our weight problems, what do we want? A quick fix. Advertise quick weight loss, and we will buy absolutely anything. Advertise quick weight loss, and we will believe absolutely everything. Outrageous statements. Ridiculous promises. Absurd testimonials. We swallow them all. Hook, line, and sinker.

"And here's the fabulous new weight loss product you've been hearing so much about, *Dr. Ima Lyer's Weight Loss Elixir.* Dr. Lyer, IMD, received her Imaginary Medical Degree from a highly respected mail-order university just last month. Her extensive research has discovered a previously overlooked medical phenomenon that causes amazingly quick weight loss.

"Dr. Lyer's Weight Loss Elixir comes in handy, single-serving-sized bottles and tastes like chocolate. When consumed at bedtime, it acts as a sleeping aid, induces lovely dreams in Technicolor, and dissolves fat while you sleep. But wait—that's not all, folks. It tightens skin, improves your complexion, and hardens your nails. Of course, there's no unpleasant exercise, and you can lose weight while continuing to eat anything you want. And we're practically giving it away! A one-month supply for the bargain price of $19.95.

"Order within the next fifteen minutes, and we'll include an additional month's supply at no extra charge. Be one of our first one hundred callers, and you'll also receive a jar of our specially formulated cellulite cream, valued at $29.95, absolutely free. In addition to reducing cellulite and eliminating stretch marks, this amazing cream removes warts and prevents hair loss. Order now. Supplies are limited."

No matter how incredible the claims, we appear to be easy prey for any and all weight loss advertising. Lose ten pounds in forty-eight hours! *You bet, sign me up.* Pills and potions that melt weight away! *Sounds great, where do I send my money?* Snake-oil salesmen are alive and well, and they're getting rich selling weight loss elixirs and magic beans.

How has everyone reached such levels of desperation? We're fat. And we're getting fatter.

Is there any other human endeavor that squanders so much time, effort, and money, and yields such wretched results as dieting? We're told that 95 to 98 percent of the weight we lose is eventually regained. This level of failure would simply not be tolerated in any other enterprise. Here in Kentucky, if diet counselors coached basketball, they'd be stoned to death.

What effect have all our diet failures had on our weight loss goals? Very little. Even though we're moving further and further away from those goals, we're simply not willing to change them. We just spend more money on promises that don't deliver results.

Ambitious Goals

No one in America is happy with their weight. No matter our present weight, we all want to weigh less. A *little* less? No. A little less is not good enough. We want to weigh a *lot* less. What is it about human nature that causes us to struggle so determinedly against being average? When I was overweight, I was stunningly overweight. But whenever I began a diet, did I pick the average female number to strive for? Of course not.

The mythical "average female" is reported to be 5'4" tall, weigh 164 pounds,[3] and wear a size 14.[4] (Or maybe a 12 or a 16 depending on the brand.) But I'm only 5'2". Since I'm shorter than the average woman, I obviously need to weigh less. Never mind that my weight was 83 pounds greater than the average woman's. When I decided to do something about it, suddenly average wasn't good enough. I hadn't weighed less than 200 pounds in ten years, yet weighing 164 pounds wasn't sufficient. Was I crazy? Yes. But I was not alone.

A recent national survey indicted that one-third of Americans are on a diet.[5] Health care professionals consider a diet successful if 5 to 10 percent of total body weight is lost, since this level of weight loss can produce statistically significant improvement in those medical conditions that are related to overweight, such as high blood pressure and type 2 diabetes.[6] The typical dieter, however, sets far more ambitious goals.

In a study of overweight women,[7] whose average weight was 220 pounds, members of the group selected 135 pounds as a *dream weight*. This represented a 38 percent reduction in body weight. Their *happy weight* was 150 pounds, a 32 percent reduction in body weight; their *acceptable weight* was 164 pounds, a 25 percent reduction in body weight. The group indicated they would be disappointed in a 10–15 percent weight loss. A 10 percent loss would be 22 pounds; a 15 percent loss would be 33 pounds.

Why would anyone be disappointed in a weight loss of 33 pounds? We're not satisfied with losing weight. We want to be thin. No matter how heavy we are, we don't want to be *less heavy*. We want to be *thin*.

What else do we want?

- We want to be thin *now*.
- We want it to be easy to *get* thin.
- We want it to be easy to *stay* thin.

When it comes to losing weight, we want instantaneous, painless, and permanent results.

Verbal Weight Loss

When we moved to Kentucky in June of 2000, I stood very calmly in the Department of Motor Vehicles and told a spectacular lie. Now, I normally consider myself to be an honest person, but one major, ironclad, cast-in-stone, no-doubt-about-it Rule of Life is that none of us tells the truth when someone asks about our weight.

We all know that we're going to lie. And the heavier you are, the bigger the lie. How many pounds can you deny without the person behind the counter breaking into hysterical laughter? I opted for a verbal weight loss of 72 pounds. The woman behind the counter put 175 pounds on my license without batting an eyelash. Bless her kind soul.

What should my license have read? Birth date: 10/18/52. Height: 5'2". Weight: 247 pounds. What did these vital statistics reveal?

- Forty-seven years old
- Short
- Fat

I didn't mind being forty-seven. I was used to being short. I hated being fat. And I was fat enough to meet the medical definition of morbid obesity, 100 pounds over normal weight.

When I was lying about my weight at the Department of Motor Vehicles, I could easily have been included in that overweight women's study. I weighed 247 pounds, and my *dream weight* coincided with theirs, 135 pounds. That weight represented a 45 percent reduction in body weight and, coincidentally, corresponded with the medical definition of normal weight for my height. I needed to lose a mere 112 pounds in order to satisfy the dream of being thin.

The justification for my lie was easy. I was starting a new diet, so it was just a matter of time before the weight on my license was correct. Perfectly reasonable, right? Based on the logic of that statement, I started thinking about the last time the weight on my driver's license was accurate.

When I was a senior in college, I gained 20 pounds my final semester. I had stupidly signed up to take organic chemistry pass/fail. I had more credit hours than I needed to graduate, but I needed a three-hour science elective. My husband, Brett, was a chemical engineering major, so I thought it would be nice if I learned a little organic chemistry. This was not a wise decision on my part, and *a little* was exactly how much I learned. By the time I survived the course, and somehow passed, I weighed 147 pounds. It was the most I had ever weighed. I would never have believed that one day I'd weigh 100 pounds more.

In the summer of 1974, I joined Weight Watchers for the first time, and I lost 35 pounds. Therefore, sometime in the fall of 1974 I would have weighed what my driver's license said I did. It had been twenty-seven years since my license weight had been correct.

The worst part of this story is that even when I weighed 112 pounds, I wasn't happy with my body. I still looked bad in shorts, because my thighs were not perfectly proportioned with the rest of my body. My fingernails hadn't miraculously become long and strong. No photographer appeared begging me to participate in a photo shoot featuring "Women of the Big Ten." I was thinner than I'd been since fifth grade, and I still wasn't happy with my body.

The Dream of Physical Perfection

The dream represents more than just being thin; the dream represents physical perfection. A great body is just the beginning. Women also want flawless makeup, and an excellent manicure, and thick, shiny, manageable hair. Men want muscular chests, and flat stomachs, and enough hair that their scalp doesn't show through. We all want to be attractive, and we're willing to consider injections, liposuction, and surgery in our search for external beauty.

Why do we do this to ourselves? Why do we insist on comparing ourselves to the limited and unrealistic images presented by Hollywood and Madison Avenue? Based on the height, size, and weight of the average woman, there has never been a greater difference between the women chosen to represent us and ourselves. And even though we know it, we still blame ourselves, rather than the people responsible for creating this disparity.

These societal influences contribute to our unrealistic expectations of appropriate weights and body shapes. Television and print ads surround us with images of disgustingly young, amazingly tall, impossibly thin women. Oh yeah, and it's not enough that they're young and tall and thin, they're also gorgeous and have high, firm, full breasts. Where do they find these women? Are they cloning them in the basements of New York modeling agencies? Are they grown on specially grafted trees in a top-secret research facility high in the Hills of Beverly?

Trust me, these women are *not* average. Remember the average woman? She's 5'4" tall, weighs 164 pounds, and wears a size 14. How does she compare to the average model? The average high-fashion model is 5'10" tall, weighs 117 pounds, and wears a size 4 or 6. The only thing that the average woman has in common with the average model is that neither is happy with their weight. They're both on a diet.

When we lose weight, we're devastated to discover that losing weight simply produces a smaller version of our less-than-perfect bodies. We can wear a smaller size. We look better in clothing. But we still look crummy in a bathing suit.

Who should we blame? Fairy stories or television or movies? Have we spent so much time looking at unrealistically beautiful people that we can no longer recognize normal? Quit watching TV. Go to the mall, to the grocery store, to the discount store. Look around. This is what normal looks like. *And normal is okay.*

Are we doomed to be shallow and unhappy? If we find a genie's bottle washed up on the beach, will we ask for thin thighs or world peace? If we catch a leprechaun perched on a rainbow, do six-pack abs seem more important than a cure for AIDS?

Focus on the Possible

If you want to lose weight and keep it off, you have to start by making changes in your head. When you decide to diet, do so with realistic expectations. Losing weight changes a number on the scales. It may make you happier and healthier; it won't make you perfect.

If you're a hundred pounds overweight, it's easy to decide that you need to lose weight. But the question is not necessarily easy to answer if you're ten, twenty, or even forty pounds heavier than the recommended weight for your height.

If you're fifty, and you're still trying to weigh what you did when you were twenty, you're expecting a lot. If you're a reasonable weight, if your blood pressure is normal, if you're not diabetic, if your cholesterol and triglycerides are in the normal range, maybe you should quit worrying about the scales and start walking for a half hour every day.

Before you decide to go on a diet, make sure that your present weight isn't okay for this age and stage of your life. If you do decide to go on a diet, focus on getting to a healthy weight and getting some exercise. Focus on what's possible.

Accept the fact that your thighs are not going to be thin. Consider the possibility that it doesn't matter. It's not only mentally unhealthy to set completely unrealistic goals, it also makes losing weight and keeping it off much more difficult.

CHAPTER 2

The Perfect Diet

Since you purchased this book, there's a good chance you're over-weight or obese and looking for help. The government keeps lots of statistics on health and nutrition, and the most recently published results have focused tremendous attention on the nation's *epidemic of obesity*. According to the National Health and Nutrition Examination Surveys (NHANES), the percentage of the population that is overweight or obese keeps increasing, from 47 percent (1976–80) to 56 percent (1988–94) to 65 percent (1999–2002).[8] In today's society, "normal weight" is no longer the norm.

In June 2000, Diane and I fit nicely into the national statistics, but we didn't fit nicely into anything else. Diane needed to lose more than 200 pounds. I needed to lose at least 100 pounds.

If I lost 100 pounds, I could move out of the Land of the Morbidly Obese into the slim, trim Neighborhood of the Merely Overweight. The loss of 100 pounds would put me at a weight of 147 pounds. This had been one of my weight plateaus (before I moved on to weight mountains). It was what I weighed at age twenty-two, when I joined Weight Watchers the first time. It was what I weighed each of the two times I became pregnant. It was the lowest weight I achieved after each pregnancy.

It was also a weight I hadn't seen in about fifteen years, but losing 100 pounds sounded nice. In fact, it sounded great. But I wanted more than just weight loss for myself. I was a morbidly obese mother with a daughter whose weight was completely out of control, and I blamed myself for her weight problems. In addition to my own excess body weight, I was also carrying around a staggeringly heavy load of maternal guilt.

Despite her weight and my concerns, Diane had always been an extrovert with many friends, and she describes her former self as "a remarkably well-adjusted person who just happened to have been really fat." She was a good student and active in extra curricular activities, but her college experience hadn't included any personal relationships. I lived with the fear that my daughter would never marry or have children of her own, because I had failed her.

While I worried about Diane's personal future, her father worried about her health. She had her gallbladder removed at age twenty, and Brett was very concerned about the serious health risks associated with her extreme obesity. And he was worried about my health as well. What could he do to help us? In the summer of 2000, he gave us a remarkable gift; he gave us the gift of time.

We were a family in transition; Brett had changed jobs, and he and I were moving from Michigan to Kentucky. Diane was graduating from college, and Brett wanted her to move with us rather than look for a job. He offered to support the two of us for an entire year so we could try to lose weight. He asked us not only to lose weight, but also to "figure out what was wrong with our lives and fix it." His goal for us was not simply weight loss, but weight loss we could maintain. His goal for us was happier, healthier, longer lives. His gift to us was the opportunity to achieve together what neither of us had been able to accomplish alone.

On June 12, 2000, Diane and I made a commitment to each other and to Brett to try *one more time* to lose weight. Who could have guessed how much our lives were going to change?

Diet Failures

What made this time different? After spending decades playing the lose-it, find-it, find-some-more game of unsuccessful weight loss, what did we do to finally get it right? First, we spent hours thinking and reading and talking about losing weight; it was our *only* responsibility. Losing weight was *our job,* and we were determined not to disappoint our benevolent employer.

Diane and I both have backgrounds in engineering, and engineers are trained to solve problems. We approached weight loss as a problem to be solved, and utilized the scientific methods we had learned in school. We started by analyzing our previous weight loss failures to determine if our past mistakes could provide a framework for future success.

If, for instance, we could identify *when* and *why* our previous diets failed, would we be able to recognize useful patterns that would help us avoid the same mistakes this time around? Suddenly, a lifetime of frustration was magically transformed into useful research.

When did our diets fail?

Sometimes the diets failed us at the beginning. They allowed so little food, or placed such extreme restrictions on the food permitted, that we couldn't stay on the diet long enough to lose any significant amount of weight. Even when we managed to lose weight by following one of these diets, we never kept the weight off long-term. Sometimes we gained it back quickly. Sometimes we gained it back slowly. But we *always* gained it back. Instead of the diet failing at the beginning, it failed at the end.

Why did our diets fail?

The diets that failed us in the beginning failed due to our *minds'* responses to our dieting choices. We were bombarded by promises of fast and easy weight loss, so we started each new diet with the same unrealistic expectations. At the beginning of the diet, when weight loss was rapid (due primarily to the loss of water), we did well. As soon as weight loss slowed, due to our bodies' natural physical reactions (more on that in chapter 4), we became discouraged and quit. We hadn't mentally prepared ourselves to make any permanent and sustainable changes in our diet.

After we determined that our previous diets had failed due to our normal psychological and physical reactions to dieting, we began to itemize the requirements of the perfect diet. The diet that wouldn't fail us at the beginning; the diet that wouldn't fail us at the end. The diet we could stay on a really long time. *The diet that would keep the weight off.*

Searching for the Perfect Diet

Now that we knew exactly what we were looking for, we began searching diligently for that perfect diet. I started at the library and at the new and used bookstores. There's a never-ending supply of diet books, so Brett and I read new ones and old ones, million-copy sellers and one-print wonders. I highlighted and took notes, and I asked Brett question after question.

What did we discover? There are lots of books, but the same information and misinformation keeps getting repackaged, recycled, relabeled, and resold. Many of the supposedly new ideas are just minor variations on old themes. And some of these old ideas were conceived when our knowledge and understanding of physiology and nutrition was tremendously limited.

Nontraditional diet books present ideas that differ from the traditional medical community's opinions on health and nutrition, and explain the conflict by indicating that *they* are privy to information the rest of the medical community is lacking. These books frequently contain elaborate explanations for *their* personal diet theory, but underneath a lot of pseudoscientific explanations designed to impress and intimidate readers, the basic rules of thermodynamics have not been changed.

Diets work when your caloric intake is less than your caloric expenditure. To lose weight, you need to burn more calories than you consume. This basic fact is frequently disguised by elaborate rules for what to eat, and when to eat it, and what to eat it with. But if you cut through the camouflage, you end up with a reduced-calorie diet masquerading as something more impressive. And frequently it's a diet that is not nutritionally balanced due to the restrictions placed on the consumption of certain food groups.

Traditional diets place no restrictions on types of foods, they simply reduce daily caloric intake in order to achieve weight loss. Since many nutrition experts believe it is very difficult to consume adequate nutrients at these caloric levels, these diets are often referred to as semi-starvation diets. Most of us have had personal experience with the accuracy of this description. It is very difficult to eat the calorie allotment of the typical reduced-calorie diet without feeling physically hungry, bodily fatigued, and mentally deprived.

When I finished analyzing our personal diet failures and studying the research about traditional and nontraditional diets, what did I conclude? If your goal is to lose weight, it doesn't matter which diet you follow.

A study of subjects following a number of popular diets determined that their daily caloric intake consistently fell in the range of 1400–1450 calories per day. Since the typical American diet contains 2200 calories,[9] following any of these diets produced weight loss.

High-fat, low-carbohydrate diets: 1414 total calories
- Dr. Atkins Diet
- Zone Diet
- Sugar Busters
- Protein Power

Moderate-fat diets: 1450 total calories
- USDA Food Guide Pyramid
- DASH (Dietary Approach to Stop Hypertension) Eating Plan
- American Diabetic Association
- Weight Watchers
- Jenny Craig

Low-fat and very-low-fat diets: 1450 total calories
- Volumetrics
- Dean Ornish's Eat More, Weigh Less
- New Pritikin Program

Look beyond the theories, discard the complex rules, ignore the complicated charts, and where do we end up? *Even when we're following a diet that theoretically does not restrict total calories, we consciously or unconsciously decrease our caloric intake.* When we're in "diet mode," we hold our daily caloric consumption to 1400–1450 calories, and we lose weight.

It's not which diet we choose, it's how long we manage to stay on it that determines whether or not we lose any weight. *Any diet that decreases caloric intake will produce weight loss.* And that decrease in caloric intake appears not to be a result of which diet we choose, but rather our own psychological response to *being on a diet*.

How do you decide which diet to follow, if you're looking for more than just weight loss? I'm always fascinated when someone who's lost weight, gained it all back, and is striving to lose the same weight again, tells how *well* they do on that particular type of diet. Excuse me. If you lose weight on a diet, but you don't maintain *any* of that weight loss, you haven't done well. Losing weight shouldn't be the sole criterion of whether or not a diet is successful.

We have all arrived, however, at a point where the long-term results of our own personal dieting experiences are so depressing that most of us no longer expect weight loss from *any* diet to be permanent. And the statistics for weight maintenance indicate that our diets are delivering exactly what we've come to expect.

Why don't our diets keep weight off? They're not designed to keep weight off. Diets are designed to make you *lose* weight. Period. And that's what they do. If you want to lose weight *and keep the weight off*, you have to do something different.

If being overweight were the problem that needed to be solved, then a diet would be the right choice. But being overweight is a *symptom* of the problem, not the problem. The problem is an unhealthy lifestyle: poor eating habits and physical inactivity. Diets try to fix the obvious symptom rather than the underlying problems. In order to achieve and maintain a normal weight, we have to fix the correct problem.

When we diet, we make temporary changes, so we lose weight temporarily. In order to lose weight permanently, we need to make permanent lifestyle changes. If you lose weight without making permanent changes in your habits, you're setting yourself up for another diet failure.

If you are slightly overweight, you can lose weight by making small changes in your habits. The heavier you are, the greater the changes you need to make in your life to achieve and maintain a normal weight. We don't need better or different diets. We need better *habits*.

In order to achieve and maintain weight loss, we need to learn how to eat like the normal-weight person *we wish to become*. We need to learn to consume a well-balanced variety of nutritious foods in the proper portions to maintain a healthy weight.

CHAPTER 3

Eucalorics

If you're overweight or obese, and you want to learn to eat correctly, how do you begin? Based on the government statistics on overweight and obesity, the School of Correct Eating appears to be closed. Or is it? If 65 percent of us are overweight or obese, and 2 percent of the population is underweight,[10] do a little math and you discover that 33 percent of the population is still managing to maintain a normal weight. What are these people eating? In my case, what is the 5'2" female who's a normal weight having for breakfast, lunch, and dinner? In order to achieve and maintain a normal weight, *I need to learn to eat like her.*

But first, I have to identify the normal weight I'm hoping to achieve. I need to know how normal weight is defined.

For many years, desirable weights were based on weight-for-height tables from the Metropolitan Life Insurance Company. The tables were gender specific and varied according to "frame" sizes defined by wrist measurements. (In the days before carbohydrate allergies, anyone who was overweight was *large-framed.* Is it possible that large-framed people are susceptible to food allergies?)

Today, the most common definitions of weight classification rely on the calculation of an individual's BMI (body mass index), and body mass indices are determined using the following mathematical formula:

$$\text{BMI} = \frac{\text{weight in pounds}}{\text{height in inches}^2} \times 704.5^*$$

*Since this formula was developed in metric units, weight in kilograms divided by height in meters squared (m²), the constant 704.5 is needed to convert the formula to English units: weight in pounds divided by height in inches squared. Depending on rounding, this constant may vary slightly. The World Health Organization uses 704.5.

What we refer to as a *normal weight* is actually a range of weights that corresponds to BMIs (body mass indices) between 18.5 and 24.9. The correlation between BMIs and weight categories is summarized in Table 3.1.

Table 3.1: Definition of BMI weight categories

BMI	<18.5	Underweight
BMI	18.6–24.9	Normal weight
BMI	25.0–29.9	Overweight
BMI	30.0–34.9	Obese I (mild)
BMI	35.0–39.9	Obese II (moderate)
BMI	40.0–44.9	Obese III (extreme)
BMI	>45.0	Obese IV (morbid)

The BMI calculations can be presented in a table, as shown in table 3.2. The range of normal weights (in pounds) for my height, 5'2", or 62", is highlighted.

If you're a power lifter, whose lean muscle to fat ratio is extremely high, or a frail little old lady, whose lean muscle to fat ratio is extremely low, the BMI calculation doesn't work very well. For most of us, however, the BMI calculations and charts give a pretty accurate assessment of our weight category.

Looking at the chart indicates that a *normal weight* for my height ranges from 101 to 135 pounds. How convenient that my previously identified dream weight of 135 pounds makes the normal-weight cut. Terrific. Now let's get to the important stuff. What do I get to eat if I want to weigh 135 pounds?

Research physiologists use a variety of formulas[11] to calculate

Table 3.2: A chart based on BMI calculations

HEIGHT	NORMAL	OVERWEIGHT	OBESE I	OBESE II	OBESE III	OBESE IV
58	88–118	119–142	143–166	167–190	191–214	over 214
59	91–123	124–147	148–172	173–196	197–222	over 222
60	95–127	128–152	153–178	179–203	204–229	over 229
61	98–131	132–157	158–184	185–210	211–237	over 237
62	101–135	136–163	164–190	191–217	218–245	over 245
63	104–140	141–168	169–196	197–224	225–253	over 253
64	108–144	145–173	174–202	203–231	232–261	over 261
65	111–149	150–181	180–219	210–238	239–269	over 269
66	114–154	155–184	185–215	216–246	247–278	over 278
67	118–158	159–190	191–222	223–253	254–286	over 286
68	121–163	164–196	197–229	230–261	262–295	over 295
69	125–168	169–202	203–236	237–269	270–303	over 303
70	129–173	174–208	209–242	243–277	278–312	over 312
71	132–178	179–214	215–249	250–285	286–321	over 321
72	136–183	184–220	221–257	258–293	294–330	over 330
73	140–188	189–226	227–264	265–301	302–340	over 340
74	144–193	194–232	233–271	272–309	310–349	over 349
75	148–199	200–239	240–278	279–318	319–358	over 358
76	152–204	205–246	246–286	287–326	327–368	over 368

Basal Energy Expenditure (BEE). (The BEE indicates how many calories we're theoretically burning, so we can know how many calories we can eat to maintain or lose weight.)

It's important to recognize that these calculations are based on best-guess estimates. The formulas may be not only gender- but also age-dependent. They're affected by our ratio of lean muscle to fat, and our exercise frequency and level of intensity. Most significantly, the calculations are based on "averages" of basal metabolic rates.

For most of us with a history of "yo-yo" dieting, there is concern that we have decreased our basal metabolic rates by subjecting our bodies to a series of self-induced famines. Additionally, numerous studies indicate that we all tend to underestimate our caloric consumption. For these reasons, we use the "low end" of caloric consumption in our calculations of daily caloric intake. We assume that an inactive female can maintain weight by consuming 12 calories per pound of body weight. (That number is based on 10 calories per pound for basic metabolic processes such as breathing and cell maintenance, and 2 calories per pound for walking to the refrigerator, pushing the buttons on the remote, and shopping for junk food.) An inactive male gets 14 calories per pound to maintain weight. (More on this obvious inequity later.) If I want to weigh 135 pounds, I calculate my daily caloric intake as follows:

$$135 \text{ pounds} \times 12 \text{ calories}/\text{pound} = 1620 \text{ calories}$$

Table 3.3 lists daily caloric allotments for both men and women based on this formula. My calculation is highlighted on the table.

Table 3.3: Daily caloric allotments by gender and weight

WOMEN									
LBS.	CALORIES	LBS.	CALORIES	LBS.	CALORIES	LBS.	CALORIES	LBS.	CALORIES
100	1200	125	1500	150	1800	175	2100	200	2400
105	1260	130	1560	155	1860	180	2160	205	2460
110	1320	**135**	**1620**	160	1920	185	2220	210	2520
115	1380	140	1680	165	1980	190	2280	215	2580
120	1440	145	1740	170	2040	195	2340	220	2640
MEN									
LBS.	CALORIES	LBS.	CALORIES	LBS.	CALORIES	LBS.	CALORIES	LBS.	CALORIES
150	2100	175	2450	200	2800	225	3150	250	3550
155	2170	180	2520	205	2870	230	3270	255	3620
160	2240	185	2590	210	2940	235	3340	260	3690
165	2310	190	2660	215	3010	240	3410	265	3760
170	2380	195	2730	220	3080	245	3480	270	3830

Using a mathematical formula produces an exact number, but it's important to remember that the calorie factor used in this formula is based on best-guess estimates of a variety of factors. *A formula based on estimates produces a result that is an estimate.* In the prose of the book, I estimate my daily caloric intake to be *about* 1600 calories, rather than the precise 1620 calories calculated by the formula.

I didn't need a daily caloric intake carved in stone; I needed a place to start. I needed to recognize that wanting to weigh 135 pounds means I have to be mentally and physically happy eating *about* 1600 calories every day. Day after day. Forever.

What did I need to do to achieve my goal of weighing 135 pounds? I needed to *practice* weighing 135 pounds. In order to weigh 135 pounds, I started eating as if I already *did* weigh 135 pounds; I started eating about 1600 calories a day.

If you're reading this book and you're female, there's a reasonably good chance that your dream weight is the same as my dream weight, 135 pounds. I'm willing to bet the following thought just popped into your head: "Sixteen hundred calories? It'll take *forever* to lose any weight. I'll just eat a little less."

Stop and take a deep breath. Remember all those diets you've been on? They haven't worked! You've lost weight, but you've always, always, *always* gained it back.

In order for this approach to weight loss to work, *you have to be willing to make one extremely significant change in the way you approach weight loss.* You *have* to quit worshipping at the altar of quick weight loss.

Advertising quick weight loss may sell diet books and a truly astonishing number of "miracle" diet pills, but it's not doing a thing for teaching us, the overweight population, how to lose weight and *keep it off.*

When people find out I've lost a hundred pounds, the first question they invariably ask is, *"How long did it take you?"*

What's my answer? "You're asking the wrong question."

Okay. What's the right question?

How long have you kept the weight off?

What possible difference does it make how long it took me to lose it, if in the process of losing it *I've learned to keep it off*?

I was an experienced participant in the weight loss game. I tried every new diet. I bought books and magazines. I knew about carbohydrate addictions and sugar allergies. I watched infomercials. I read about zones and counting points, and, despite all my efforts, I'd spent the last twenty years getting fatter and fatter. And I'd passed my weight problems on to my daughter.

Diane started having serious weight issues when she was quite young, and she was much heavier at age twenty-two than I had ever been. When people find out that we've lost this much weight without having bariatric surgery, they can hardly believe it. And, of course, they want to know how we did it.

So we tell them about the basis for Eucalorics.

Eucalorics isn't about losing weight quickly. It's about losing weight forever! It's about accepting responsibility for your present weight problems and learning to make permanent changes in your life that will allow you to achieve and maintain a healthy weight.

Accepting Responsibility

No one wants to be overweight, but as we struggle and fail at losing weight, we're easily seduced by any explanation that allows us to blame our obesity on factors that are not in our control. Best-selling diet books are filled with elaborate theories for why we're over-weight. They tell us we eat the wrong types of food, we eat the wrong combinations of food, we eat incorrectly for our blood type, we me-tabolize insulin improperly, or we eat at the wrong time of day.

Has it helped us to blame our weight on someone or something other than ourselves? Not a bit. Before we can solve our weight is-sues, we have to identify the source of our problems, and we need to start by admitting some unpleasant truths. Why is everyone fat? Because we eat too much and exercise too little.

Yuck. We hate that answer.

You want a different answer? Okay.

Why is everyone fat? Because our caloric intake is greater than our caloric expenditure.

That's not fair. It's the same answer. It's just dressed up a little to be polite.

Sorry. If you want a different answer, buy a different book. There are lots to choose from. When we typed "diet/health/fitness" into the search engine at Amazon.com, there were more than 30,000 books in the database. These books are filled with scientifically complicated but polite explanations for overweight. In these books, *other* dieting theories are difficult, but once you understand *their* particular theory, dieting is supposed to be easy.

In real life, when you put the book on the coffee table and walk into the kitchen, the reverse is true. Theoretical dieting may be easy, but actual dieting is hard. It's time to stop dieting and start learning to eat. It's time to learn new habits.

The first critical step in learning new habits is admitting the truth about our old habits. Why were we fat? We didn't have metabolic disorders, and we weren't allergic to carbohydrates. Our thyroids were functioning, and our pancreases were doing a fine job producing insulin. Why were we fat? We were victims of overactive fork disease, and our tennis shoes never played tennis. We ate too much and exercised too little.

When do we lose weight? When our body's energy equation is unbalanced. What does this equation look like?

caloric intake = base metabolism + physical activity = caloric expenditure

When our bodies are in a state of caloric equilibrium, our caloric intake equals our caloric expenditure, and we maintain weight. If our caloric intake is less than our caloric expenditure, we lose weight. We're eating an insufficient number of calories and/or exercising. If our caloric intake is greater than our caloric expenditure, we gain weight. We're eating an excessive number of calories and/or practicing for a career as a couch potato.

Each pound of stored fat represents 3500 calories of potential energy. In order to lose a pound of fat, we have to be calorically "out of balance" by a deficit of 3500 calories. Our caloric intake has to be 3500 calories less than our caloric expenditure. Since caloric expenditure is a combination of basic metabolic processes and exercise, we can lose weight by reducing caloric intake, increasing our exercise level, or both.

If we do not make *sustainable* changes in our eating habits and physical activity levels while losing weight, we have very little chance of maintaining that weight loss.

What's the best way to create new habits? *Practice new habits.* Do the same thing over and over.

If you want to be a specific weight, calculate how many calories it takes to maintain that weight. Start eating that number of calories. Every day. Day after day. Forever.

Stop worrying about losing weight quickly. Start concentrating on losing weight forever by learning new eating habits.

People with weight problems know how to diet. We know how to overeat. We know how to starve. We know how to binge. We don't know how to eat normally.

Eucalorics is based on the premise that weight loss should occur as a result of eating the number of calories that will support a healthy weight. Eucalorics isn't a traditional diet that requires semi-starvation caloric intake to achieve weight loss; Eucalorics isn't a nontraditional diet that relies on complicated rules about what to eat or when to eat. Eucalorics is a weight maintenance program. Maintenance starts the first day. Weight loss happens while you're practicing maintenance.

When you reach your goal weight, weight loss stops. You keep practicing maintenance. One day you look around and you're not practicing maintenance anymore, you're just maintaining.

CHAPTER 4

A Different Approach

People ask us about weight loss all the time. Lose three hundred pounds and, trust me, people get very interested. We give them the same embarrassingly easy explanation we gave you.

Pick a weight. Calculate how many calories it takes to support this weight. Start eating that number of calories. Don't stop.

How do they respond?

It seems *too easy* to be a real diet. It seems *too sensible* to be a real diet. We're so used to restricted calorie or restricted food group diets that we don't know how to eat anymore.

Remember the definition of Eucalorics? *Eu-* means "normal"; a *eucaloric* diet is a *normal-calorie diet,* designed to achieve and maintain a healthy weight *by consistently consuming the number of calories that support that weight.* (The *eu-* is pronounced as if it were the word "you." Think of it as *you-calorics*—it puts *you* in control of your caloric intake.)

When we start a typical diet, we switch from normal eating mode to diet eating mode. The rules of diet eating are easy. If you like it, you can't have it. If it tastes good, you can't have it. If it's on a menu, you can't have it. What do you eat when you're on a diet? Grilled chicken. Lettuce. Meals in cans. Frozen dinners. Why is it so hard to stay on most diets? YOU'RE ALWAYS HUNGRY. If you try to lose weight on a traditional semi-starvation diet, you're going to be hungry.

Why did counting calories become so unpopular? It became associated with low-calorie diets (LCDs) and very-low-calorie diets (VLCDs). People came to associate counting calories with being hungry all the time following semi-starvation diets that didn't provide long-term results. These diets restrict calories in order to maximize the rate of weight loss, but *extremely restrictive diets are interpreted by the body as evidence of famine.* Since the body does not distinguish between self-induced famine and the real thing, it responds to low-calorie diets by decreasing the body's energy requirements and protein stores by reducing muscle mass.

As the metabolic rate decreases, it becomes increasingly more difficult to lose weight, despite the low caloric intake. People are literally starving themselves, and their bodies are responding by going into survival mode and burning fewer calories. Then, once dieting stops and normal eating resumes, the weight gain is accelerated because the metabolic rate is still decreased. Even worse, during the dieting phase, the body has lost muscle mass. When weight is regained it's in the form of fat that metabolizes fewer calories than muscle, so the dieters' previous weights are now sustained by fewer calories. The dieters gain back more weight than they lost, and are both heavier and have a greater percentage of body fat than when they started the diet.

Medically supervised diets have focused on the low-calorie diets (LCDs) and very-low-calorie diets (VLCDs). The low-calorie diets have people routinely consuming 1000 to 1200 calories per day, but it's *impossible* to be happy eating this number of calories. Why? There's actually a pretty simple explanation. Do a little math, and the reason becomes obvious; you're not eating enough food.

What weight does 1000 calories a day support?

$$\text{Female:} \quad \frac{1000 \text{ calories}}{12 \text{ calories/pound}} = 83 \text{ pounds}$$

$$\text{Male:} \quad \frac{1000 \text{ calories}}{14 \text{ calories/pound}} = 71 \text{ pounds}$$

No wonder you're hungry. If you're female, you're only eating enough calories to support an 83-pound woman; if you're male, you're only eating enough calories to support a 71-pound man.

If you're on a very-low-calorie diet, such as a muscle-sparing protein supplement diet, it may provide as few as 600 calories a day, and the numbers are even worse.

What weight does 600 calories a day support?

$$\text{Female:} \quad \frac{600 \text{ calories}}{12 \text{ calories/pound}} = 50 \text{ pounds}$$

$$\text{Male:} \quad \frac{600 \text{ calories}}{14 \text{ calories/pound}} = 43 \text{ pounds}$$

You're only eating enough food to support a *50-pound* woman or a *43-pound* man! Gee, no wonder your body thinks the famine has arrived. It has. No wonder your metabolic rate is decreasing— your body is trying desperately to reduce your energy requirements.

Why can't we stay on a diet long enough to lose any significant amount of weight? We're starving. I don't want to weigh 83 pounds. Why am I *practicing* to weigh 83 pounds?

We don't need to learn to diet. We need to learn to eat correctly. Eating 1000 calories a day isn't eating correctly. Eating correctly is eating a well-balanced, nutritional variety of foods that will support a healthy weight.

How do you sabotage the Eucalorics approach? You pick a weight that requires permanently subsisting on the semi-starvation rations provided by a low-calorie or very-low-calorie diet. When you decide to pick a goal weight, give yourself a fighting chance. You're allowed to pick a dream weight, but you need to stay away from fantasy weights.

What's the difference?

A dream weight is possible. It may be a long way away, it may be ambitious, but it's possible. A fantasy weight requires a plane crash on a remote desert island.

There are numerous other charts, graphs, and calculations that are used to establish desirable weights other than BMI. For some reason, it's difficult for us to resist picking the system that places us at the lowest possible weight. My fantasy weight system allows 100 pounds for the first five feet of height, and 5 pounds for each additional inch of height. According to that calculation, I should weigh 110 pounds.

There's obviously been at least one day in my life when I weighed 110 pounds, but I have no idea which day it was. Maybe it was only part of a day. Maybe I was an infant. Still, I love the idea of weighing 110 pounds. There's just one question. Which limb am I willing to sacrifice to do so?

No matter whether we try to lose weight by following a low-calorie or very-low-calorie diet or by following one of the popular food-restricting diets, we *always* set ourselves up for failure by striving for unattainable goals.

Still need to be convinced? Let's use that BMI calculation, and do a little math. (Don't panic, we'll do the math for you.)

$$BMI = \frac{\text{weight in pounds}}{\text{height in inches}^2} \times 704.5$$

Let's use this formula and take a look at the people in New York City and Hollywood that we keep comparing ourselves to. How much do the people in New York City and Hollywood get to eat?

What about the high-fashion model, remember her? She's unbelievably tall: 5'10". She's incredibly thin: 117 pounds. What's her BMI?

$$\begin{aligned} BMI &= \text{weight in pounds} \div \text{height in inches}^2 \times 704.5 \\ BMI &= 117 \div 70^2 \times 704.5 \\ &= 117 \div 4900 \times 704.5 \\ &= 0.024 \times 704.5 \\ &= 16.9 \end{aligned}$$

Her BMI is significantly less than 18.5; at 117 pounds, she's clearly underweight. Let's put this in perspective. What would I have to weigh to have a BMI of 16.9? We start with the BMI formula, then solve for weight in pounds.

$$\begin{aligned} BMI &= \text{weight in pounds} \div \text{height in inches}^2 \times 704.5 \\ \text{Weight in pounds} &= BMI \div 704.5 \times \text{height in inches}^2 \\ &= 16.9 \div 704.5 \times 62^2 \\ &= .024 \times 3844 \\ &= 92 \text{ pounds} \end{aligned}$$

Good grief, I'd have to weigh 92 pounds to have a BMI of 16.9. I think I last weighed 92 pounds in the third grade. What would I get to eat in order to maintain that weight?

$$92 \text{ pounds} \times 12 \text{ calories/pound} = 1104 \text{ calories}$$

Suppose I somehow arrive at a weight of 92 pounds. (I've been locked in a closet for eight months and fed two crackers and bottled water once a day by a crazed fashion magazine cameraman.) When I escape from the closet, I get to gorge myself on 1100 calories a day for the rest of my life in order to maintain my new weight. What can I eat with those 1100 calories?

Even if I'm very careful, it's difficult to fulfill my basic nutritional requirements on 1100 calories a day. If I'm not careful, it's easy to be out of calories very quickly. If I start my day with a large hot chocolate made with whole milk and whipped cream, I've started the day with 580 calories. Add a butterscotch pecan scone for 520 calories, and I've suddenly arrived at 1100 calories, and it's not even lunchtime.

Or I can start my day with a diet Dr Pepper, and save all those calories for later. Perhaps I'll order a low-calorie chicken Caesar salad for lunch. When I blithely consume the butter-drenched croutons and 2 ounces of full-fat dressing, that "low-calorie" salad suddenly totals 590 calories, and the 3-ounce chunk of baguette adds another 210 calories. Since I've *only* had a salad for lunch, it's perfectly reasonable to finish off the meal with a single cookie. How many calories can one cookie possibly have? Oops, that innocent-looking shortbread cookie has 340 calories. Lunch just topped out at 1140 calories.

Hmmm. Ninety-two pounds is not looking good.

Okay. I'm actually eight inches too short to be a high-fashion model. What if I'm willing to settle for becoming a star of the stage and/or screen? (We'll be polite and ignore my age.) Most Hollywood stars have heights and weights that classify them as underweight, a BMI less than 18.5. I'm willing to be a rather plump star, so I'm going to aim for a BMI of exactly 18.5.

$$
\begin{aligned}
\text{Weight in pounds} &= \text{BMI} \div 704.5 \times \text{height in inches}^2 \\
&= 18.5 \div 704.5 \times 62^2 \\
&= .026 \times 3844 \\
&= 100 \text{ pounds}
\end{aligned}
$$

What do I get to eat, if I weigh 100 pounds?

$$100 \text{ pounds} \times 12 \text{ calories/pound} = 1200 \text{ calories}$$

Wait. That number sounds familiar. Oh yeah. I've tried eating 1200 calories a day; it is the high end of the semi-starvation diet. I was *miserable* eating 1200 calories a day.

Remember my fantasy weight? A hundred and ten pounds, right? We already established that I'm *never* going to weigh 110 pounds. It simply isn't going to happen. If I'm never going to weigh 110 pounds, does it make sense for me to try to diet by eating the number of calories that sustains a weight *even lower* than my fantasy weight? A weight that I will never reach or maintain?

But that's exactly how most diets work. Most diets reduce daily caloric intake to significantly less than it takes to maintain our goal weights in order to promote quick weight loss. We're hungry, and we're miserable, because we're trying to exist on the calories that will maintain unreasonable weights.

What's the result? Either we don't stay on the diets long enough to lose much weight, or if we do lose weight, we gain the weight back. We haven't made any long-term changes to our eating habits, so we don't know how to maintain our weight loss once we get there. The diets either fail us at the beginning or fail us at the end.

I decided that the weight of a model or a Hollywood starlet shouldn't be my goal. Maybe it shouldn't be your goal. Remember, *these people are not the norm*. Do yourself a favor and pick a reasonable goal. Don't doom yourself to failure by selecting a BMI goal for which 2 percent of the population qualifies. Pick a reasonable goal. It can always be changed.

When we started, although I *wanted* to lose 100 pounds, my first intermediary goal was the 47-pound loss that would get me below 200 pounds. As the concepts that became the basis of Eucalorics evolved, days became weeks and weeks became months. At some point, I realized that the 100–pound weight loss was actually going to occur. I didn't know when it would happen. I simply knew that it *would*. And as I was losing weight, I was watching Diane lose weight too.

At her heaviest, Diane could no longer be weighed on the average physician's scale that weighs up to 350 pounds. She had so much weight to lose that she didn't bother to pick a goal weight; instead, she simply focused on getting through each day. One day at a time. When months became years, Diane had lost 200 pounds following a eucaloric diet.

What else has happened in our lives?

I don't have to feel guilty about Diane's future anymore. She's engaged to a great guy (who's an engineer), and there's nine yards of satin in the basement waiting to become a wedding dress. And invitations ready to be stuffed and mailed.

Every day, we talk to people about losing weight with Eucalorics. I get to see the absolute amazement on someone's face when they realize that it's possible to eat well and lose weight. When someone who's been struggling with her weight for years looks at me and says with wonder in her voice, "I could eat like this forever," I get to answer her, "I know." And I do.

As you continue to read about Eucalorics think about setting reasonable goals. If you're extremely obese, maybe you should follow Diane's example. Worry about where you're headed later, and start by simply trying to eat correctly one day at a time. If you're obese, begin with the goal of becoming overweight. If you're overweight or lose enough weight to become overweight, you can decide to aim for a normal weight. Keep in mind that you have to be mentally *and* physically happy eating the number of calories that will support the weight you have chosen.

I picked as a goal the highest weight that would still place me in the normal weight category. One hundred and thirty-five pounds was a dream weight, not a fantasy weight, and it corresponded to eating about 1600 calories a day. Since careful food choices and preparation made that a reasonable amount of food, Diane and I both used this number for our daily caloric intake.

The meal plans in part 2 are designed to provide 1600 calories per day; additional calories are added according to a schedule provided in chapter 15. If you happen to be a female with a goal weight of 135 pounds, you won't have to make any changes to the meal plans. Otherwise, you'll need to make some adjustments to these basic plans to reach *your* recommended daily caloric intake.

How did Diane and I achieve our present healthy weights? We stopped dieting and started eating.

CHAPTER 5

New Habits

The goal of a Eucaloric diet is not simply weight loss; it's permanent weight loss. Permanent weight loss can only be achieved
by making permanent changes in our daily fare, our diet. How do
we make permanent changes in our daily fare? We learn new habits.

The solution to bad eating habits is different than the solution to
most other bad habits. The message for most bad habits is simple.
Stop. If you smoke, stop smoking. If you bite your fingernails, stop
biting them. If you drink to excess, stop drinking. If you have a drug
problem, stop taking drugs. The cure for most bad habits is to stop
the problem behavior completely.

Diets are the equivalent to the stop solution to a bad habit. Stop
eating carbohydrates. Stop eating protein. Stop eating fat. Stop eating. But the stop solution doesn't work for food, because not eating
is not compatible with continued life and health. Bad eating habits
require change. Bad eating habits need to be replaced with good eating habits, and the key to developing new habits is repetition.

As long as my caloric consumption *averages* 1600 calories a day,
I won't gain weight. I *could* eat 800 calories one day and 2400 calories the next day. I would maintain my weight, but I would not be
developing good eating habits. The best way to learn new eating
habits is to eat consistently. Eat the same number of calories every
day. The more consistently you eat, the more habitual this new pattern of eating will become. When we eat correctly and consistently,
our bodies get used to eating the correct number of calories in the
proper portions. I've changed not only *what* I eat, but also *how* I

eat. I try to eat consistently, because eating consistently makes it easier to eat correctly.

What about losing weight?

One of the most difficult things for us is to convince people that they can lose weight while eating well. Everyone believes that losing weight means eating horrible nasty food and being hungry *all the time*. Especially if you're counting calories!

If you are overweight and begin to eat correctly, you will begin to lose weight. The heavier you are, the more quickly you will lose weight. If you exercise, you will lose weight even more quickly. In June 2000, I weighed 247 pounds. How many calories did it take to maintain that weight?

$$247 \text{ pounds} \times 12 \text{ calories/pound} = 2964 \text{ calories}$$

My instinctive reaction to that number was a quick side trip into the Land of Denial. There was *no way* that I was consuming almost 3000 calories per day. Or was I? My usual fast-food feast consisted of a batter-dipped and fried chicken breast with dressing on a bun. It was accompanied by French fries, a medium chocolate dairy dessert, and, of course, a diet drink.

Chicken sandwich	430 calories	14 fat grams
Medium fries	440 calories	20 fat grams
Dairy dessert	440 calories	11 fat grams
Total	1310 calories	45 fat grams

If I'm trying to weigh 135 pounds, I just ate 81 percent of my daily calories for lunch.

What about my personal favorite food, ice cream? It's packed in cartons whose small print mentions something about four servings. Yeah, right. My all-time favorite, chocolate chip cookie dough, has 1080 calories and 68 grams of fat in each carton, and I *never* picked up a pint without eating the entire carton. And that pint of ice cream was frequently consumed with a package of cookies.

Why was I so out of control? I had two equally unhealthy approaches to food. I was either dieting or I was *planning to diet*. And what was I doing when I was planning to diet? I was eating. No, not just eating. **EATING.**

How did I maintain my previously svelte 247 pounds? I spent a great deal of time *planning to diet.* And when I was planning to diet, I was eating pints of ice cream, and two-pound bags of chocolate, and boxes of assorted cookies. I was always planning for the period of deprivation scheduled to arrive on Monday, but the truth was that I spent much more time *planning to diet* than I ever did *dieting.*

I decided to consider the possibility that I really was averaging almost 3000 calories per day. Since I was eating that many calories each day, I didn't have to reduce my calories to starvation level in order to lose weight.

When I was eating 1200 calories a day, I was losing weight. When I started eating 1600 calories a day, I *still lost weight.* Would I have lost weight more quickly on 1200 calories a day? It depends. When I started eating 1600 calories, I was getting more food, so I *stayed* on the diet. Let's look at the numbers.

Weight loss eating 1200 calories
2964 calories/day − 1200 calories/day = 1764 calories/day
3500 calories/pound ÷ 1764 calories/day = 1.98 days/pound
7 days/week ÷ 1.98 days/pound = **3.5 pounds/week**

Weight loss eating 1600 calories
2964 calories/day − 1600 calories/day = 1364 calories/day
3500 calories/pound ÷ 1364 calories/day = 2.6 days/pound
7 days/week ÷ 2.6 days/pound = **2.7 pounds/week**

Not too surprisingly, weight loss is more rapid on a semi-starvation diet, but the difference is less than a pound a week. Am I willing to exchange a pound a week in weight loss for 33 percent more food? You bet I am. Especially since I rarely stayed on a low-calorie diet long enough to lose any meaningful amount of weight. Especially since the feelings of deprivation associated with a semi-starvation diet usually led to bingeing behavior and weight gain.

If you begin to consistently eat the calories that will support your goal weight, you will discover how much easier it is to eat sensibly when you aren't hungry all the time. It's easier, but it is still difficult to eat correctly in today's world.

In order to eat correctly, you need to become an educated consumer. The more knowledge you possess, the better the food choices you can make. You need to know as much as possible about food processing and preparation. You need to understand the psychology that influences your choices. You need to be prepared.

You're about to start making permanent changes in the way you eat. Permanent changes in the way you view food. Is it possible? Yes. Is it easy? Not always. Is it worth the effort? Absolutely.

I had spent most of my adult life unhappy about my weight and miserable around food. I didn't control my eating; my eating controlled me. Every Monday morning I started another diet. And every time I started and failed, I was miserable. Food was the one aspect of my life over which I seemed to have no control, and I hated it.

Eucalorics gave me the control. Learning to eat correctly gave me the ability to deal with my own personal "diet demons," the foods that I ate to excess, the foods I binged on. The foods that I associated with diet failure.

The frustrations associated with yo-yo dieting have warped our attitudes toward food. Food is no longer viewed as the provider of either simple nourishment or gastronomic pleasure, but as an all-powerful entity with a combination of abstract and human characteristics. It is viewed as good or bad. It is labeled legal or illegal.

Diane and I learned to accept that food is simply food. That no one comes to arrest us if we eat a cookie. An open bag of chocolate is not a sign of deep moral decay. Bad food is the food in the back of the refrigerator with mold growing on it, or chicken salad with mayonnaise sitting overnight on the counter.

Eating correctly does not focus on fat-free food or carbohydrate-free food; eating correctly focuses on guilt-free food. There are no bad foods. There are no illegal foods. Some foods are low-fat and low-calorie. Some foods are high-fat and high-calorie. It's all just food.

When any food is labeled "bad," it's human nature to instantly want it. When we begin eating these "bad" foods, we don't just eat, we binge. We eat until the bag or box is empty. As long as there is "bad" food around, we are subject to continued temptation. In order for us to be restored to *good* behavior, the bad food must all be consumed. The knowledge that *all* food is permitted appears to be a critical element in eliminating the feelings of guilt that frequently initiate and accompany bingeing. This thought is accompanied by the following valuable information: It is highly unlikely that any food available today will not still be available tomorrow. It is not necessary or recommended to try to eat every piece of candy or all of the cookies today. They'll make more.

I have lost a tremendous amount of weight, but the weight loss is *not* the best thing that happened. Somewhere along the way, I learned to eat two cookies from a package that contained twenty cookies. I learned to eat two cookies today, and two cookies tomorrow, and two cookies the next day. When you eat the box two cookies at a time, you get to enjoy eating cookies *without feeling guilty about eating cookies*. This is a big deal. When was the last time you ate cookies without feeling guilty? Since I went on my first diet when I was eleven, I had probably eaten my last guilt-free cookie when I was ten.

The ability to accept food as just food is important in developing a healthy relationship with it. It is more important to have learned to eat two cookies than to have lost weight, because learning to eat two cookies is what makes maintaining my weight loss possible. I've lost weight before. I never learned to eat two cookies before.

I am sincerely and intensely devoted to oatmeal raisin cookies, and potato chips, and every form of chocolate, and good-quality ice cream. I am willing to learn to eat them in reasonable amounts, but I'm not willing to do without them. If you learn to eat the proper portions, you can eat anything.

You need to learn to live with food, not without food, in order to lose weight permanently!

I was raised in a house with very little junk food. Did I grow up to make nutritious choices as a result? No, I grew up to be completely out of control around any high-fat, high-sugar food product, because I'd never been taught to eat it in appropriate amounts. And I did the same thing to my own children.

One of our fundamental diet truths is that there's great psychological satisfaction in getting to eat the "whole" thing. Although it's now *possible* for me to eat two cookies from a bag that contains twenty cookies, I'm still happier when I get to eat an *entire* package. This package happens to be a single-serving-sized package, but it's still my very own package, and I get to eat it *all*. Do I waste time feeling guilty about this admittedly warped attitude toward food? No. I accept that my psyche has permanent "scars" from my years of dieting; I identify my personal "warp zones" and work around them.

I'm just crazy about Nabisco's new Ritz Chips. They come in either a nine-ounce bag or in a box with twelve three-quarter-ounce bags that have 100 calories each. It's probably less cost-effective to buy the small bags, but I'm not simply purchasing the chips; I'm also purchasing a little bit of willpower. Do I occasionally eat more than one small package in a single sitting? Yes. But I've never eaten more than two. And I'd have to eat *all twelve* small bags to equal the calories in the one large bag.

There's an enormous selection of food that is presently available in single-serving sizes. The original concept may have been snack items for children's lunchboxes, but there may be a much greater market for overweight adults. Single-serving packages provide a little extra physical barrier that helps us control our eating.

I suspect that people who've never been fat don't need this type of help. Diane's fiancé has never had a weight problem, and it's interesting for Diane to watch him eat. He automatically eats reasonable portions; it's simply not a problem for him. It makes absolutely no difference to him if the cookies are in a single-serving package or in a cookie jar. He eats a single serving without having to think about it.

If the cookies are in a cookie jar, I may eat a single serving, but it's not automatic. I *still* have to make a conscious effort to eat correctly. Will it ever become automatic? Maybe. Maybe not. But it gets easier every day.

We all need to identify our own limitations. Don't feel bad if you need more help than someone else. Take advantage of anything and everything that helps *you* succeed in learning new habits. I did every-thing I could to help me learn to eat correctly, because learning to eat correctly has given me the tools to be in control. Learning to eat correctly has given me a fighting chance to maintain my weight in a world that is making everyone fatter.

CHAPTER 6

Nutrition 101

Before you read any further, it's a good idea to decide why you're unhappy with your present weight. Why do you want to change it? In order to determine what adjustments you're willing to make in your present diet, you have to decide not only *what* you want, but also *why* you want it. You've decided *how much* you want to weigh. But what does that weight represent? Do you want to be a normal weight or do you want to be healthy?

It's possible to maintain a weight of 135 pounds by eating little chocolate doughnuts. As long as you consume no more than 1600 calories per day, a little-chocolate-doughnut diet will maintain a weight of 135 pounds. But it won't be a good diet. It won't be a healthy diet.

It's possible to be a normal weight without being healthy; it's possible to be healthy without being a normal weight. Our family did more than just lose weight. We made changes in our eating habits and our lives that made us thinner *and* healthier.

In order for us to be healthy, our diets have to include the micronutrients—the vitamins and minerals—as well as appropriate amounts of the *calorie-containing* macronutrients—the carbohydrates, proteins, and fats. If we are to become thinner *and* healthier, we need to make good food choices. How do we decide what's a good food choice? We need to know something about the basics of good nutrition.

Before we get started, however, let's have a heart-to-heart about this chapter. If you've read other diet books, the nutrition chapter is the one that would be voted "Most likely to be skipped." It's the chapter that's rather scientific and fairly boring. Most of us have little interest in Nutrition 101, and we don't spend our leisure time reading textbooks.

We live in the "information age," where the media takes pages and pages of boring scientific information and distills it down to a snippet to be used as an interesting sound bite. The problem is that the interesting sound bite may not correctly summarize those pages and pages of boring scientific information. It's difficult to take complex information and make it not only easier to understand, but also interesting, and still have it be accurate.

There's a lot of information about basic nutrition floating around in media sound bites that's not completely accurate. We'd like your basic nutrition information to be accurate. In order to make this as painless as possible, we've kept the chapter short, and there won't be a test at the end.

Since the macronutrients are the *calorie-containing* nutrients, we should probably start this section by talking about calories. After all, this book is **Calorie Queens**. You may vaguely remember hearing that "a calorie is the unit of energy equal to the amount of heat required to raise the temperature of 1 kilogram of water by 1°C at 1 atmospheric pressure." Trust me, you won't need to remember or understand this definition in order to count calories.

What *do* you need to know about calories?

Food provides the energy that our bodies need to function, and *calories measure how much energy a food contains*. Carbohydrates and proteins are energy sources that provide approximately 4 calories of energy per gram of weight when converted into glucose and metabolized; fats provide approximately 9 calories of energy per gram of weight. Fats are considered energy-dense, since they contain more than twice as many calories per gram as carbohydrates or proteins.

I'd love to pretend that calories don't count, but I didn't lose 100 pounds until I was willing to admit that they do. Diane didn't lose 200 pounds until she was willing to admit that they do. If you don't want to take our word for it, get a copy of the *Dietary Guidelines for Americans 2005*. The executive summary contains the following statement: "poor diet and physical inactivity, resulting in an energy imbalance (*more calories consumed than expended*), are the most important factors contributing to the increase in overweight and obesity in this country." (The italics are mine.)

If calories are the only things that count, why do low-carbohydrate diets work?

People on low-carbohydrate diets are losing weight, but, as discussed in chapter 2, they're losing weight because they've reduced their daily caloric intake. It's true that they're not eating carbohydrates, but they're losing weight because they're eating fewer calories, not due to the lack of carbohydrates.

Diane and I lost weight while eating carbohydrates. Everyone else losing weight following our eucaloric diet is losing weight while eating carbohydrates. If you consider life without bread to be a sad life indeed, then this is really good news.

Carbohydrates

The word "carbohydrate" is so popular that it has a nickname: "carb." And carb's new best friend is "low." "Low" and "carb" are seen absolutely everywhere. You'd think a food group that gets so much press would be better understood. But, it's not. If "carb" ever decides to dump "low," it's definitely going to need a new marketing team.

This fine and upstanding member of the body's macronutrient team has been transformed into the demon-spawn food group by the "it's not our fault we're fat" ad agency. The problem is that the carbohydrate food group not only includes the whole grains, fruits, and vegetables that our body needs to be healthy, it also includes the vast majority of the "junk food" we eat. It's not the high-quality carbohydrates we need to eliminate from our diets; it's the non-nutritious junk food.

When you hear the word "carbohydrate," don't think low, think plant. Carbohydrates are products that are directly or indirectly derived from plants. Since fruits and vegetables are plants, *fruits and vegetables are carbohydrates*. If this is the only thing you get out of this chapter, you're already a step ahead, because everybody else still thinks that carbohydrates are just bread and potatoes.

What else should you know about carbohydrates?

If you're on a scavenger hunt and the first three things on your list are monosaccharides, disaccharides, and polysaccharides, you don't need a chemical supply store, you need a grocery store. These *saccharides* are the three categories of carbohydrates that are present in the foods we eat every day.

The most basic carbohydrates are the *monosaccharides*, also known as the simple sugars: glucose, fructose, and galactose. They're simple sugars not because they're stupid, but because the body breaks down *all* carbohydrates into these three simple sugars. The liver then turns fructose and galactose into glucose, and the cells use glucose for energy. Glucose and fructose are found in fruits, vegetables, corn syrup, and honey; galactose is created when milk sugar is digested.

The second classification of carbohydrates is the *disaccharides*, the double sugars. The best-known sugar, sucrose, is a disaccharide. It's the sugar that comes in five-pound bags and, in Kentucky, makes tea really sweet. It comes from cane, beet, and maple sugar, and we're all eating lots of it. Maltose, familiar to beer drinkers as malted barley, and lactose, milk sugar, are the other disaccharides commonly found in food.

The third classification of carbohydrates is the *polysaccharides*, commonly referred to as the complex carbohydrates, which may be composed of thousands of long strands of simple sugars. This long-strand structure allows the complex carbohydrate to be broken down slowly, providing energy in a *time-released* form.

These complex carbohydrates are found in foods as either starches or fiber.

Starches include the cereal grains (wheat, rice, and corn); legumes (peas and beans); and root vegetables (carrots and potatoes).

Fiber is cellulose, cannot be digested, and may be either soluble or insoluble. Soluble fiber assists with normal digestion, and reduces blood cholesterol levels. Insoluble fiber, commonly known as roughage, aids in digestion by reducing the occurrence of constipation, and may help protect against colorectal cancer. There are also indications that fiber may help to reduce blood pressure levels. In addition to these specific health benefits, the presence of fiber in diets adds bulk and helps satiate us after a meal.

WHY DO WE NEED CARBOHYDRATES?

Carbohydrates are the main source of our body's preferred form of energy: glucose. Glucose is the primary energy source for the central nervous system; the brain cannot survive without blood glucose, so carbohydrates are brain food.

SIMPLE VERSUS COMPLEX CARBOHYDRATES

There is tremendous confusion regarding the difference between simple carbohydrates and complex carbohydrates. *Any* carbohydrate that is not a simple or double sugar is a complex carbohydrate. White rice, brown rice, white flour, and whole wheat flour are *all* complex carbohydrates. White rice and white flour are simply more processed than brown rice and whole wheat flour.

Whole grains contain all three parts of the grain kernel: the bran, the endosperm, and the germ. Removing the fiber and B-vitamin-packed bran and germ during the milling process, leaving only the endosperm behind, produces white flour. When the bran and germ are removed, the grain becomes less nutritious, but it's still a complex carbohydrate.

Proteins

Unlike the carbohydrates, the protein food group has a great marketing team. In today's low-carb world, carbohydrates are the bad guys, and proteins are everyone's favorite food group. The high-protein, low-carb diets insist that the body digests proteins differently, and everybody ignores the fact that most people are eating "proteins" that are actually *combination foods* containing as much or more fat as protein.

The body breaks down or metabolizes the dietary protein we eat into amino acids. These amino acids become the building blocks that are recombined to produce the more than 100,000 different proteins found in the body, proteins that are composed of only twenty different amino acids in an amazing variety of combinations. Our bodies can synthesize eleven of these amino acids; the remaining nine, known as the essential amino acids, must be supplied by our diet.

When you hear the word "protein," you probably think animal, but proteins originate from both plant and animal sources, and dietary proteins are not all created equal.

If you consume dietary proteins that originate from animal sources, you are eating *complete* proteins, proteins that contain all the essential amino acids. Eggs, milk, cheese, meat, poultry, and fish contain complete proteins.

The proteins derived from most plant sources, however, are *incomplete* proteins, proteins that do not provide all nine of the essential amino acids. Cereals, legumes, nuts, and vegetable proteins are all incomplete proteins. Certain combinations of incomplete plant proteins can be combined, however, to produce all essential amino acids. Rice and beans is a classic example of a *complementary* protein relationship.

Ingestion of complete or complementary dietary proteins is key to maintaining health. If a specific amino acid needed to construct a particular protein is not available, the protein will not be made. There are no substitutions for essential amino acids. If a diet is lacking in a specific amino acid, the function of every protein in the body that contains that amino acid will be affected.

Despite the "eat all you want" mentality associated with the high-protein, low-carb diets, the body has a very limited capacity to store amino acids. Once proteins are metabolized into amino acids, any excess amino acids are either converted to glucose and stored as glycogen in the muscles or the liver or are converted directly to fat.

WHY DO WE NEED PROTEIN?

Proteins are responsible for all body tissue growth, repair, and maintenance. The body's hormones and enzymes, as well as the antibodies our immune system uses to fight disease, are proteins. Proteins play a vital role in the structure of all body cells and in the regulation of body processes, and when our glucose stores run low they provide an alternative source of energy. The muscles in our bodies account for more than half the body's protein, and protein is normally contained in every tissue and fluid in the body with the exception of bile and urine.

Fats

Fats used to have the marketing team that's presently working for the carbohydrates. The 1990s were the fat-free decade. As long as you never ate anything that had more than 30 percent fat, it was supposed to be easy to be thin. But the '90s came and went, and we didn't become thin.

Fats also originate from both plant and animal sources, and plant sources generally produce unsaturated fats. Unsaturated fats are often liquid at room temperature. Vegetable oils such as corn, peanut, and safflower, as well as avocados, hazelnuts, and almonds all contain unsaturated fat.

Saturated fats, such as butter or lard, are solid at room temperature, and are usually associated with animal foods. Since much of the saturated fat we consume is a component of the proteins we eat, reducing the fat in our diet can be complicated. Eggs, cheese, cream, bacon, chicken, and beef all contain saturated fats.

WHY DO WE NEED FAT?

Fat is a necessary part of our diet because of the important roles it plays in our bodies. While the carbohydrates we eat are our main energy source, our body's fat is our built-in energy reserve. Fat is a source of, and acts as a carrier for, the fat-soluble vitamins A, E, D, and K. Fat is also a major component of cell membranes. Why does everyone care about how much and what types of fat we're consuming?

When your doctor sends you down to the lab, they draw blood and run a blood lipid profile. When he looks at the results and starts lecturing you about triglycerides and cholesterol, he's fussing about the amount and type of fat cruising around in your bloodstream. The fat in your diet shows up not only on your waist and hips, but also in your blood vessels, your vascular system.

When do you get fussed at? When you have a higher percentage of low-density lipoproteins (LDLs) in your profile; the LDLs are the *bad guys*. (This is about the only time when "low" is a bad thing.) Lipoproteins are the class of proteins that transport fat throughout the body, and they are classified according to their fat to protein ratio. Since fat is less dense than protein, a lipoprotein that is composed of more fat than protein has a lower density; it's a low-density lipoprotein (LDL).

Conversely, since protein is more dense than fat, a lipoprotein that has more protein than fat has a higher density; it's a high-density lipoprotein (HDL). The HDLs are the *good guys*.

WHY SHOULD YOU CARE?

When the fat the body needs to function is being transported through the bloodstream in LDLs (the low-density lipoproteins), the cholesterol in the LDLs ends up being deposited in the walls of blood vessels, causing atherosclerosis, "hardening" of the arteries. Strokes and heart attacks are associated with this type of blood vessel disease, since it is more difficult to pump blood through these narrowed, hardened vessels.

Generally, the unsaturated fats from vegetable oils are considered *good* fats, because they increase the levels of high-density lipoproteins in the blood. The monounsaturated oils, such as olive oil and canola oil, are better choices than the polyunsaturated oils.

Saturated fats from animal products are generally considered *bad* fats, because they increase the levels of low-density lipoproteins in the blood. Hence the recent emphasis on cooking with vegetable oils such as olive oil or canola oil rather than with butter.

For many years, it was assumed that *any* dietary fat from a *plant* product was more healthy than *any* dietary fat from an *animal* product. As a result, margarine and shortening were considered to be healthier choices than butter. Margarine and shortening, however, are manufactured products, created by a process known as hydrogenation.

During hydrogenation hydrogen atoms are added to normally unsaturated vegetable oil. The hardness of the resulting product varies depending on the amount of saturated fat produced. One by-product of hydrogenation is trans-fatty acids, and recent studies suggest that the effects of trans-fatty acids on blood lipid (fat) levels are similar to those of saturated fat.

At the same time the trans-fatty acids, which are derived from a plant product, began to receive bad reviews, the omega-3 fatty acids, which are present in animal products, began to get positive reviews. Omega-3 fatty acids are found in cold-water fish, especially the fatty varieties like albacore tuna, herring, salmon, mackerel, sardines, and anchovies, as well as some leafy vegetables, seeds, and oils.

In 1971, Danish researchers discovered a link between the omega-3–rich diets of Eskimos living in Greenland and their low rate of cardiovascular disease. The omega-3 fats appear to improve atherosclerosis by removing cholesterol from the walls of arteries. Additional research suggests that these types of fatty acids may also help protect us against cancer and rheumatoid arthritis.

Eating the proper types and amounts of fats, combined with daily exercise, can improve your blood lipid profile substantially, and decrease your risk of heart disease and stroke.

No matter the source of the fats in our diet, there is little argument that the typical American diet contains more fat than recommended. Most dietary guidelines suggest that no more than 30 percent of total calories should come from fat, with no more than 10 percent from saturated fat.

The American Heart Association, American Cancer Society, and American Medical Association, as well as the federal government's nutrition policies, all endorse a diet that yields no more than 30 percent of your calories from fat, and no more than 10 percent from saturated fat.

But when we walk into a store, we don't buy a carbohydrate; we buy bread. We don't buy protein; we buy cheese. In order to translate the macronutrients into daily life, we need to look at the foods that comprise a healthy diet.

CHAPTER 7

Making Changes

What kind of changes can you make in your eating habits that will result in permanent changes in your life? The heavier you are, the more changes you need to make. You have to start somewhere; where's the sensible place to start? The U.S. Department of Agriculture (USDA) and the Department of Health and Human Services' (HHS) Food and Drug Administration (FDA) are the government agencies responsible for the federal nutrition policies. These agencies issue the most well-known recommendations for nutrition and health, the *Dietary Guidelines for Americans*. The original guidelines were issued in 1980, and new guidelines are issued every five years. The most recent set was issued in January 2005.

The eighty-page report can be summarized in ten words:

- Eat fewer calories.
- Be more active.
- Make wiser food choices.

This chapter addresses the nutrition recommendations embodied by the "make wiser food choices" portion of the dietary guidelines.

There's always tremendous debate surrounding these seemingly innocuous and sensible guidelines, and much of that discussion focuses on their "food choice" recommendations. Controversy centers on the conflict between promoting *health* or promoting *business* that any adjustment in nutrition policy inevitably provokes. There is intense lobbying and pressure from special interest groups, and critics maintain that these groups detrimentally influence the specific wording of the dietary guidelines.

I'm prepared to let the professionals argue about the nuances of word choice. I'm willing to concede that these dietary guidelines are not perfect. It's hard for me to believe, however, that the average American diet would not be significantly improved by following these admittedly imperfect guidelines.

Diane and I are not, and do not pretend to be, registered dietitians or nutrition professionals. And although Brett can certainly provide medical opinions and explanations, I decided that many of our decisions regarding nutrition require more common sense than academic training. And having been morbidly obese qualified Diane and me to address some of the "get real" aspects of the present American diet and make sensible recommendations to change it.

In some ways, not being a professional makes it easier. I don't have to give the professional line or politically correct answer. I can provide the "give me a break" answer. I'm not obligated to tell you what you should do; I'm allowed to acknowledge what you're going to do. I don't have to encourage perfect choices; I can get excited about better choices. I live in the real world, not in an ivory tower.

The professionals are arguing about insufficient emphasis being placed on the benefits of eating brown rice rather than refined white rice. Excuse me, please. The average fat person is eating *fried* rice.

They don't want me to eat a plain baked potato with chili on it because potatoes have a high glycemic index? Haven't they noticed that I'm surrounded by people eating super-sized orders of fries?

Would we be better off eating whole grain bread products? Certainly. And if we're in the process of fine-tuning an already excellent diet, then whole grains are not only the best choice, they're also a remotely possible choice. But if today's breakfast was biscuits with sausage gravy and a side of hash browns, isn't hoping for wheat berry toast with soy butter a trifle optimistic?

Just as I believe that losing weight by subsisting on starvation rations is doomed to failure, I have similar reservations about making sudden and drastic changes to our present diets. Macrobiotic diets should probably be shelved next to fantasy weights. When we're picking out unreasonably low numbers for our scales, we're contemplating food choices we normally wouldn't feed the hamster.

If your present diet is a veritable banquet of high-fat, high-sugar choices, don't decide to go cold turkey on junk food on the first day. It's easier and less stressful to make gradual changes to your diet. If you've been a fast-food aficionado, now is not the time for heroic changes. Start by adding fruits and vegetables to your diet. You can always add bulgur and tofu later.

My previous diet was not a healthy diet, and there's a good chance that your present diet looks like my old diet. Why are we doing so poorly? Surveys about diets indicate that most people are overwhelmed by the amount of information available. As a result of the *epidemic of obesity,* the media gives significant airtime to issues concerning overweight and obesity, but today's message may not agree with yesterday's message. And confident, well-spoken individuals with impressive letters after their names delivered both messages. How do we decide whom to believe?

We used a commonsense approach to dietary choices. We looked at the recommendations one category at a time. What looked reasonable? If one set of recommendations didn't seem possible, we didn't throw up our hands in frustration and walk away. We did what we could. And we kept improving our diet by continuing to make gradual changes in our daily fare. And we keep improving it.

We keep trying to expand our fish consumption, and Diane is working to develop recipes that incorporate more legumes (beans) into our diets.

The new dietary guidelines were released on January 12, 2005. What are we supposed to be eating? (Serving sizes are based on recommendations in the DASH Eating Plan for 1600 and 2000 calories.)

Grains

1600-calorie eating plan: 6 servings
2000-calorie eating plan: 7–8 servings
Serving size: 1 slice bread
        1 ounce dry cereal
        ½ cup cooked rice, pasta, or cereal

We've all been eating lots of grains, but we've been eating them in highly processed, high-fat, high-sugar, and high-calorie snack food. Instead of whole grain toast, we're eating doughnuts. Glazed doughnuts? No, chocolate-covered, cream-filled doughnuts.

This new set of guidelines specifies that at least half of our grain choices should be whole grain. Walk down the bread or cereal aisle at the grocery store and you can easily identify the power of these new guidelines on the food industry. Products labeled "whole grain" are everywhere.

Will these new guidelines make that much difference in our diets? When the bold print on the front of a cereal box declares, "Made with whole grains," but the back of the box still reads, "Less than 1 gram fiber per serving," it's hard to get very excited about this "improved" product. The dieticians would prefer to see the total sugar decrease and the fiber increase.

Why are we supposed to eat whole grains, anyway? A lot of the reason is fiber. If you eat your fruits and vegetables, you'll get lots of fiber. If whole grain bread and brown rice aren't in your future, but you eat lots of fruits and vegetables, you won't have to feel as guilty about eating white bread. Do what you can. The goal is to improve.

Want some good news? Popcorn is considered a whole grain product. I buy the 94 percent fat-free microwave popcorn, and I often eat it as my evening snack. Oatmeal is a whole grain; I eat oatmeal. I'm even thinking about eating brown rice. Diane is not.

Fruit

> 1600-calorie eating plan: 4 servings
> 2000-calorie eating plan: 4–5 servings
> Serving size: 6 ounces fruit juice
> 1 medium fruit
> ¼ cup dried fruit
> ½ cup fresh, frozen, or canned fruit

Most of us are not consuming the recommended amounts of fruit, and six fruits—orange juice, bananas, apple juice, apples, fresh grapes, and watermelon—account for nearly half the fruit consumption in this country. In order to improve, we need to eat more fruit, and we need to eat a greater variety.

Since most of us like fruit, it's not hard to add fruit to our diet. It makes a good morning or afternoon snack. Or start substituting fruit for those heavy and fattening desserts.

Vegetables

1600-calorie eating plan: 3–4 servings
2000-calorie eating plan: 4–5 servings
Serving size: 1 cup raw leafy vegetable
    ½ cup cooked vegetable
    6 ounces vegetable juice

In the vegetable group, the recommendations also specify weekly intake from each of the five vegetable subgroups:

- Dark green vegetables (3 cups/week)
- Orange vegetables (2 cups/week)
- Legumes (3 cups/week)
- Starchy vegetables (3 cups/week)
- Other vegetables (6½ cups/week)

Vegetables are the category of food we're all supposed to eat, but we don't. In my previous life, my attitude toward vegetables was simple: I didn't eat them. I ate salads, but the greens were drowning in full-fat dressing. I ate potatoes, but the potato was loaded with butter, sour cream, and bacon. Now I eat vegetables.

I eat asparagus and sugar snap peas; I eat stewed tomatoes and okra; I eat broccoli and cauliflower. I'm totally and completely amazed at what I eat. What do I want you to do? Give vegetables a chance.

Remind yourself that Diane and I didn't eat vegetables before and now we do. Look at our pictures and consider the possibility that vegetables are responsible for this amazing transformation. You've been willing to try almost anything to lose weight, haven't you? How bad could eating a few vegetables be compared to some of the things you've tried?

Here are the rules:

- If it's covered with cheese, it doesn't count as a vegetable.
- If it's swimming in a cream sauce, it doesn't count as a vegetable.
- Potatoes, corn, and peas count as starches, not vegetables.

What's left? Look at the menus in part 2. Every dinner has a vegetable. Remember the 300 pounds? I started by adding baby carrots as an afternoon snack. They come in a small package, don't need to be washed, don't require a utensil, and don't need to be cooked. Pretend they're not good for you, and it should be easy to add them to your diet.

Meat

1600-calorie eating plan: 1–2 servings
2000-calorie eating plan: 2 servings
Serving size: 3 ounces cooked meat, poultry, or fish

Americans get much of their protein from red meat, and most of that red meat protein is in the form of ground beef. We include recipes that use ground beef in this book, but we only use the lowest-fat version of ground beef available: 96 percent extra-lean ground beef. We also eat a great deal of pork, but we only use the leanest cuts of pork: the center cut of the pork loin or the pork tenderloin.

Why use these lower-fat products? Fewer calories. Less fat.

We eat lots of chicken; the recipes in the book use primarily boneless, skinless chicken breasts. We also eat fish and seafood. Chicken, fish, and seafood are naturally lower in fat and saturated fat than red meat products.

We had one gentleman who ate dinner with us for twelve weeks, and at the end of that twelve weeks had lost 27 pounds. He was pleased with his weight loss, but he wasn't willing to continue eating our dinners. He was a "meat and potatoes" guy, and our meals were just a little too different for him to handle.

If you're struggling with your weight, and you've spent your life eating red meat and potatoes, now might be a good time to consider expanding your culinary horizons.

Low-Fat or Fat-Free Dairy Foods

1600-calorie eating plan: 2–3 servings
2000-calorie eating plan: 2–3 servings
Serving size: 8 ounces milk
1 cup yogurt
1½ ounces cheese

This set of guidelines specifies low-fat and fat-free dairy products. If you're trying to decrease the fat content of the dairy products you normally consume, make gradual changes.

If you normally drink whole milk, start drinking 2 percent. If you normally drink 2 percent, start drinking 1 percent. If you normally drink 1 percent, start drinking skim.

Drink a lower-fat version for three or four weeks. Choose the next-lower-fat product and repeat the process until you're drinking skim. I mixed 1 percent and skim for three weeks.

Don't whine about it. Nobody likes to listen to a whiner. Just ask Diane. (Yeah, I did a lot of whining about skim milk.) I was convinced that I would *never* get used to drinking skim milk. But I did.

Why drink skim milk? Why eat low-fat sour cream and cottage cheese? Fewer calories. Less fat.

Fats & Oils

The fat recommendations for the DASH Eating Plan are extremely low. (The USDA Food Guide allows twice as much fat.)

1600-calorie eating plan: 2 servings/week
2000-calorie eating plan: 2–3 servings/week
Serving size: 1 teaspoon soft margarine
1 tablespoon low-fat mayonnaise
2 tablespoons light salad dressing
1 teaspoon vegetable oil

The fat in our diets comes not only from fats and oils, but also from the fat in meat and dairy products. If we are not careful, fat sneaks into our diets.

Switch to the low-fat and skim versions of dairy products and the extra-lean versions of beef and pork, and you'll not only improve your diet's caloric content, you'll also greatly improve its fat content.

Sweets

The sweets recommendations for the USDA Food Guide place sweets in a category labeled "discretionary calories." You'll notice that the 1600-calorie eating plan includes *no* calories for sweets (a rather unrealistic recommendation).

> 1600-calorie eating plan: 0 servings/week
> 2000-calorie eating plan: 5 servings/week
> Serving size: 1 tablespoon sugar
> 1 tablespoon jelly or jam
> ½ ounce jelly beans
> 8 ounces lemonade

We're all eating lots of sugar. Our increased consumption of snack foods has not only reduced our consumption of fiber and complex carbohydrates, but also has helped skyrocket our consumption of added sugar.

Why should you care about added sugar? Sugar supplies calories without nutrients and fiber. It's instant energy that the body doesn't have to do any work to get. If you have a limited number of calories, sugar displaces healthier alternatives.

Sodium

Due primarily to concern about the relationship of salt intake to hypertension, the dietary guidelines recommend consuming less than 2300 mg of sodium per day. (That's approximately one teaspoon of salt per day.) The vast majority of the salt we consume is introduced by food manufacturing. If you rely on food prepared by others, it can be difficult to lower your sodium. Using low-sodium chicken broth can greatly improve a recipe's nutrition profile, and this product is specified in several of our recipes. Just as you can "train" yourself to eat and drink lower-fat milk products, you can also decrease your taste for salt. As we have prepared more and more of the food we eat, I have become much more sensitive to the flavor of salt. We previously used the regular version of soy sauce; we now use only low-sodium soy sauce, and I find even the lower-salt version to taste extremely "salty."

As I lost weight, I made gradual but significant changes in my eating habits. My present diet bears little resemblance to my previous diet, and I am continually amazed at the transformation that has occurred. I would never have believed it was possible to make this dramatic a change in my diet at this point in my life. But it was.

Because of the changes I have made, I am now mentally and physically happier with my daily caloric allotment. Do I eat perfectly? No. But, I consistently make better food choices, and my head and my body are content with my present diet.

CHAPTER 8

The Big Bad World of Food

You've learned a little nutrition. You've taken a look at the recommended servings for your daily caloric intake. You're ready to make some changes in your imperfect diet. Out the door you go into the real world. A world filled with food.

Food is everywhere. Walk the aisles at the grocery store on a Saturday afternoon, and it's possible to consume a meal's worth of calories in free samples: a new variety of cookie, a slice of deli cheese on a cracker, a little piece of pizza, a taste of cheesecake. And it's not just the grocery store. There are chocolate coins at the bank, mints by the restaurant cashier, and toffees at the dry cleaners.

The U.S. food industry is presently producing 3900 calories per day for each and every man, woman, and child in America. After adjusting for wasted calories, such as leftovers, spoilage, and oil used for frying, that number becomes 2800 calories per day.[12]

What happens if you're female and you consistently consume *your share* of this abundance of available food? If the food supply creates 2800 calories a day *just for you,* and you eat it, what will you weigh? Remember the 12 calories per pound calculation?

$$\frac{2800 \text{ calories}}{12 \text{ calories/pound}} = 233 \text{ pounds}$$

What if you're male?

$$\frac{2800 \text{ calories}}{14 \text{ calories/pound}} = 200 \text{ pounds}$$

Where do all these calories go? To our waists, to our hips, to our thighs. What's the inevitable result of this abundance of calories? We're all fat. We're all fat, because we're surrounded by food. All the time. Everywhere we go. And what kind of food are we surrounded by? We're surrounded by junk food.

Junk Food

What is *junk food*? It's the high-sugar, high-fat, high-sodium, high-calorie food that provides little or no nutrition. It's eaten while standing or driving; it's eaten when bored or upset. It's eaten without regard to the calories it contains. It's the readily available, rapidly consumed, and quickly forgotten food that packs amazing amounts of calories in remarkably small packages. There is calorie and nutritional information on each and every bag of chips and bar of chocolate, but it could be printed in hieroglyphics for all the attention it receives.

While our minds are ignoring the calories that junk food contains, our waistlines and hips are paying attention. And junk food is available everywhere. It's at the checkout line in every conceivable type of store. Whether you're purchasing copier paper, or a hammer, or three yards of lace, you can walk away from the cash register with chocolate in your chubby little fist.

Junk food is easy to eat. It doesn't need to be washed; it doesn't need to be peeled or chopped. It doesn't require a knife or fork, or any pots and pans, or an oven, or a microwave. It's quickly transformed from potential calories in a package to extra inches on your thighs, and this transformation is occurring every day, everywhere, to everyone.

The results of this omnipresent banquet of junk food are diets that contain too few vitamins and minerals, and too many calories. According to an analysis of data from the 1999–2000 National Health and Nutrition Examination Survey (NHANES), almost 25 percent of our calories are eaten in the form of sweets and desserts, soft drinks, and alcoholic beverages. Add another 5 percent from salty snacks and fruit-flavored drinks, and *30 percent* of our total caloric intake is coming from nutrient-poor food.[13] And poor nutrition is only the beginning.

ENERGY DENSITY

In addition to having a poor nutrition profile, junk food is generally energy-dense; it's high in calories, but low in volume. Energy-dense food represents maximum calories in minimum space.

If we're trying to maintain a healthy weight, eating energy-dense foods means we don't get to eat very much. And the less food we consume, the less likely that our bodies will feel full and satisfied with the number of calories that support our selected weight.

Studies show that the weight of food people consume is more constant than the calories they consume.[14] If you eat the same amount (by weight) of food, but lower the average calorie density, you will consume fewer calories but still feel satisfied. The high percentage of junk food in our diets, however, is having the opposite effect. The high energy density of most junk food makes it very easy to eat excessive amounts of calories.

Junk food is packed with sugar by a variety of names. The label may say sugar, sucrose, glucose, fructose, maltose, lactose, dextrose, invert sugar, raw sugar, honey, molasses, brown sugar, barley malt, date sugar, turbinado sugar, cane sugar, maple sugar, caramelized sugar, distilled or concentrated fruit sugars, or corn syrup. It's all sugar. Instant energy. Calories without nutrients.

Even though carbohydrates provide only 4 calories of energy per gram of food, a "fat-free" snack food, such as a jelly bean, is very energy-dense because it's *all* sugar. Let's compare the energy-density of two carbohydrates: a 4-ounce apple and 4 ounces of jelly beans. Both are a high-sugar snack, but the apple contains fiber and water in addition to fructose (the natural sugar found in fruits), so its energy density is significantly less than that of the jelly beans.

A four-ounce apple:

$$\frac{67 \text{ calories}/4 \text{ ounces}}{28 \text{ grams}/\text{ounce}} = 0.60 \text{ calories}/\text{gram}$$

Four ounces of jelly beans:

$$\frac{416 \text{ calories}/4 \text{ ounces}}{28 \text{ grams}/\text{ounce}} = 3.71 \text{ calories}/\text{gram}$$

The apple has an energy density of 0.60; the jelly beans have an energy density of 3.71. The energy density of the jelly beans is more than six times the energy density of the apple. If you've allotted about 70 calories to an afternoon snack, you can either have a small apple or *seventeen* jelly beans. And the seventeen jelly beans do not contribute fiber, vitamins, or minerals to your daily fare.

Fruits and vegetables (particularly vegetables) are low-energy-dense foods. But it's possible to alter the intrinsic energy density of any food by varying its preparation. The primary culprit? The ever-popular deep-fat fryer. What effect does frying have on energy density? Let's look at a high-fiber, low-calorie, complex carbohydrate: the potato.

An ordinary baking potato with skin has approximately *20 calories and 0 grams of fat per ounce.*

Now, cut that same potato into six wedges, introduce them to a deep-fat fryer, and suddenly the baked potato becomes cottage fries that have *70 calories and 4 grams of fat per ounce.* If you prefer thin fries, it's easy to reach *90 calories and 5 grams of fat per ounce.* Slice the potato paper thin, and the all-American potato chip arrives at *150 calories and 10 grams of fat per ounce.*

Variations in food preparation have increased the potato's calories per ounce data, from 20 calories per ounce to 150 calories per ounce. What effect did preparation have on the potato's energy density? The greater the surface areas in contact with the oil, the higher the energy density and the higher the calories.

Plain potato:

$$\frac{20 \text{ calories}/\text{ounce}}{28 \text{ grams}/\text{ounce}} = 0.71 \text{ calories}/\text{gram}$$

Potato chips:

$$\frac{150 \text{ calories/ounce}}{28 \text{ grams/ounce}} = 5.36 \text{ calories/gram}$$

The plain baking potato has an energy density of 0.71; our potato chips have an energy density of 5.36. The energy density of the chips is nearly *seven and a half times* higher than the energy density of the baking potato.

Why should you care? Because it means that you can eat seven and a half times as much baked potato as potato chips for the same number of calories. Since you have a limited number of calories to consume to maintain a healthy weight, you can either eat energy-dense foods and be hungry *all the time,* or you can choose your daily fare more carefully and be physically and mentally happy with your diet.

In order for our bodies to be *happy* with the caloric intake that maintains a normal weight, we need to be *smart calorie consumers.* We're all smart shoppers. We look for sales. We search out bargains. We recognize the value of the good deal. We need to apply our sharply honed shopping skills to the world of food. We need to start recognizing the *good deal* foods. These are the low-energy-dense foods that maximize the amount of food we can eat without maximizing the number of calories we're consuming.

Where do you find these good deal foods? Grab that shopping cart and head for the fresh food section. The high-fiber, high-water-content vegetables are the big winners in the "eat more, weigh less" food contest. The recipe for Roasted Asparagus (p. 130) makes six 3-ounce servings. You could eat all six, be positively stuffed, and only have eaten 150 calories. Vegetables help fill you up without filling you out.

If I can only eat 1600 calories a day, I want those to be the best-tasting, most flavorful calories I can find. Highly processed foods contain sugar, salt, fat, and natural and artificial flavorings that are added to compensate for the nutrients and flavor removed by the processing procedures. Low-nutrition, low-fiber, processed foods provide *expensive* calories that do not make my body happy with the volume of food it has received. But it is particularly difficult to avoid snacking in today's world.

DOES IT MAKE THAT MUCH DIFFERENCE?

It can. It is very easy to add 200–300 calories to your day by consuming a single candy bar. I picked up a chocolate bar at the grocery store yesterday to look at the nutritional information. My favorite candy bar would add a quick 280 calories to my caloric intake. If I'm already consuming the amount of calories that I'm balancing by physical activity, what does the addition of a daily candy bar do to my weight?

$$\frac{3500 \text{ calories/pound}}{280 \text{ calories/day}} = 12.5 \text{ days to gain a pound}$$

$$\frac{365 \text{ days/year}}{12.5 \text{ days/pound}} = 29 \text{ pounds/year}$$

I haven't allowed any calories for digestion, so that number is not completely accurate, but it's still a pretty scary number. It demonstrates that it doesn't take very many extra calories to gain weight.

If you've become fairly casual about picking up "a little something" to tide you over until dinner, and you don't adjust dinner to compensate for those extra calories, snacking could be one explanation for some of your weight problems. If you're a tall male who can eat 2600 calories a day, it's easier to find calories for snacking. And it's not as critical for those snacks to be nutritious. If you're a petite female, you don't have many extra calories to spare. If you want to be the correct weight, and eat a healthy diet, it's difficult to find room for junk food.

THE MONTH OF CANDY MADNESS

My previous diet was filled with junk food. And it wasn't easy to give it up at first. The first Halloween after we started dieting was October 2000. We had been dieting for approximately four months when the snack-sized candy bars appeared at the grocery store. Each bar contained about 50 calories. An easy and attractive size for a snack. We bought a bag.

We were initially very pleased with ourselves. We carefully noted the calories consumed each day in chocolate. We never binged. We were doing so well, it seemed safe to have more than one kind available, so we bought another bag. We never exceeded our daily caloric allotment, but the number of calories assigned to chocolate kept getting bigger. And neither one of us wanted to admit what was happening. Eventually, I was up to 400 calories in chocolate, 25 percent of my daily calories. And I was hungry, because the energy-dense chocolate didn't provide enough food for the calories it contained.

We dubbed it the Month of Candy Madness, and it hasn't been repeated. It was our first lesson in the power of energy density, and it gave birth to the concept of the saturation of the senses: the idea that the first bite tastes best.

Saturation of the Senses

There is medical evidence that all senses become saturated. Smells are strongest when first detected. Water feels hottest at the first touch. Does excessive eating also saturate our taste buds? If it does, then the first bite actually does taste best. If the product is not wonderful, it will not improve by continued consumption. If we keep eating until the bag is empty, all we will accomplish is emptying the bag. If the first bite doesn't provide the proper level of mouth pleasure, we'll never get it by consuming more.

Some of the best-tasting food is served as hors d'oeuvres—single bites of intense flavors. Tasting menus provide small portions of multiple courses. Expensive wines are sampled by swirling a single taste in the mouth. Are all these examples of the unnoticed fact that the first bite tastes best?

Is overeating an unconscious effort to re-create the intense flavor associated with that first mouthwatering bite? If you eat only the best food you can, and you pay attention to what you eat, and you savor *every* bite, it's much easier to be satisfied with the proper portions of food.

How can you exist in this world of caloric abundance and maintain a normal weight? You're already taking the first step. The first step is recognizing the cause and the extent of the problem. Once you acknowledge the severity of the problem, you can start learning to coexist with this ubiquitous supply of food. In order to control how much food you're eating, you have to pay attention. You have to play an active role in deciding what goes in your mouth.

Learning to eat correctly is not a spectator sport!

We're overweight and obese, because the world in which we live makes it easy to be fat and difficult to be thin. It's possible to lose and maintain weight by learning to eat correctly, but being a healthy weight still requires self-discipline.

The heavier you are, the more likely it is that your diet has included a significant number of calories from high-energy, high-calorie, and low-nutrient food. If you're trying to not only maintain a normal weight, but also consume a healthy diet (one that contains the recommended ratios of carbohydrates, protein, and fat, and appropriate levels of vitamins and minerals), most of your daily caloric allotment is used up fulfilling the basic nutritional needs. *The fewer calories it takes to maintain your desired weight, the fewer discretionary calories your diet contains.* And junk food calories should come from your discretionary calories; the calories left over after all the nutritional calories have been consumed.

It's not necessary for every morsel of food that crosses your lips to be healthy. It's not reasonable to expect that you'll never eat junk food again, but it's important to become extremely selective with those discretionary calories. When I decide to eat an energy-dense food, I make sure it's worth the calories it contains.

I would personally consider a life without chocolate to be a miserable existence indeed. But I no longer pick up a candy bar at every checkout line I pass through. When I decide to eat chocolate, I eat a reasonable amount. And I only eat really good chocolate.

If I'm at the mall, I sometimes head to the Godiva kiosk. I'll spend several minutes carefully perusing the truffle selection. Then I'll purchase one truffle, and eat it *slowly*. And enjoy it. The rule about junk food is simple: Eat within your discretionary calories, and *don't feel guilty* when you're eating it. I no longer waste the calories that maintain a healthy weight on mediocre food, junk or otherwise. But junk food is allowed, it's just not allowed all the time.

CHAPTER 9

High-Maintenance Eating

I read lots of books on dieting, and I was fascinated by the books that told me to listen to my body to know when I was full. My amused reaction was, *Excuse me, you obviously haven't noticed that I'm a hundred pounds overweight?* (Okay, okay, maybe a hundred and ten.) If I knew when my body was full, I wouldn't be in this shape. I didn't rely on internal signals to tell me when I was finished eating. I relied on external signals.

When are we finished eating? When the bag is empty. When our plate is clean. When the cupboard is bare. When are we finished eating? We're finished *when the food is gone.*

If you are tremendously overweight, you have been abusing your body for years; your stomach no longer sends the appropriate "I'm full" signals. The *goal* is to be able to listen to your body. But first, your body needs help. Your body needs to be consistently fed correctly, until it learns how much food you should be eating. Your mind and your body need to be taught how a proper portion of food looks and tastes.

If you want to achieve and maintain a normal weight, you have to be a *high-maintenance eater.* You have to be willing to pay attention to the food that goes in your mouth. Not only *what* you're eating, but also *how much* you're eating.

If you decrease the amount of junk food in your diet, it will become easier to eat the number of calories that maintain your healthy weight. But you need to be aware that the body stores *all excess dietary calories* as body fat. When it comes to storing excess calories, the body is an equal opportunity storage facility.

If you're eating excess *carbohydrates,* the body converts those excess carbohydrates into body fat and stores it. If you're eating excess *protein,* the body converts that excess protein into body fat and stores it. If you're eating excess dietary *fat,* the body converts that excess dietary fat into body fat and stores it.

Are we noticing a pattern here?

If you are consuming more calories than your body is using for basic metabolism and physical activity, those excess calories are stored as body fat. *It doesn't matter where those excess calories come from.* Even a diet that contains absolutely no junk food can contain too many calories due to excessively large portions of *nutritious* food.

Improving our diets, our daily fare, involves more than simply changing what we eat. We also have to be aware of how much we eat. We have to know not only what constitutes a serving, but also how many servings support a specific weight. The more calories it takes to support a normal weight, the more servings or larger portions can be consumed.

There's also the calorie factor to be considered. Since men have a higher calorie factor (14 instead of 12) than women, it takes more calories for a male to support *the exact same weight.*

If you're a female with a goal weight of 150 pounds, it takes 1800 calories per day to maintain that weight.

150 pounds × 12 calories/pound = 1800 calories

If you're a male with the same goal weight, 150 pounds, it takes 2100 calories to maintain that weight.

150 pounds × 14 calories/pound = 2100 calories

The man has a caloric advantage of 300 calories per day. Where does this outrageously unfair advantage come from? Muscle mass.

Men's bodies average 22 percent muscle; women's bodies average 15 percent muscle. Even if a woman and a man are the same height and the same weight, the man gets to eat more food to sustain that weight than the woman, due to his greater muscle mass. Muscle burns more calories than fat, so the natural tendency of men to have a higher muscle mass means they can eat more calories than a woman of identical height and weight.

The average man is also taller than the average woman. Since height is one of the factors in the BMI calculation, the average man can weigh more than the average woman due to his increased height, and still have a normal weight as defined by the BMI calculations.

The realities of weight are particularly harsh, therefore, for someone like me. I'm a 5'2" female. With whom shall I register my complaint? My mother who is 5 feet tall or my grandfather who was 5'4"? When I sit down to dinner with just about anyone, male or female, they're going to get to eat more than I do. If you're female, it's particularly hard to be thin. If you're a short female, it's even harder. You simply don't have very many extra calories to play with.

If I had only been a little overweight, it would be easy to blame my weight problems on my height and my gender. But I wasn't a *little* overweight. I was morbidly obese. My weight was the result of eating excess calories of all varieties. How many *extra* calories was I eating? How many *extra* calories are you eating?

What did my numbers look like?

247 pounds × 12 calories/pound = 2964 calories
135 pounds × 12 calories/pound = 1620 calories
2964 calories – 1620 calories = 1344 calories

Fill in your numbers on the next page.

What did my 1344 extra calories represent? Easily available calories. When I paid no attention to making good food choices, to food preparation, or to caloric content, I averaged 2964 calories per day, and 1344 of those calories were the difference between being morbidly obese and being a normal weight.

The heavier you are, the more *extra* calories you're consuming. If most of your meals are eaten away from home, a significant number of those extra calories are the result of unreasonable portion sizes. When we eat out, we relinquish control. And in the modern

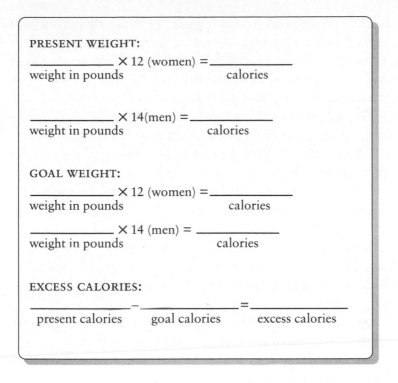

PRESENT WEIGHT:

_____ × 12 (women) = _____
weight in pounds   calories

_____ × 14(men) = _____
weight in pounds   calories

GOAL WEIGHT:

_____ × 12 (women) = _____
weight in pounds   calories

_____ × 14 (men) = _____
weight in pounds   calories

EXCESS CALORIES:

_____ − _____ = _____
present calories   goal calories   excess calories

world of meals outside the home, a variety of complex social and economic factors influence the meals and portions we receive.

If you're trying to be healthy while eating out, there are usually about three choices on the menu that appear remotely possible. One of them is grilled chicken, and the other two sound nasty. You order the grilled chicken and a salad, and you end up feeling sorry for yourself. The next thing you know, you're having the chocolate brownie à la mode to make yourself feel better.

Have big should a portion be? How many calories should it contain? It depends. Who's going to eat this meal? Short, inactive, older females should be consuming smaller amounts of food than growing adolescent males. The caloric intake *should* be a function of height, weight, and activity level of the diner. In the restaurant business, however, these decisions are based on economic considerations.

How do we get you into our restaurant? How do we maximize the amount of money you will spend? And how do we get you to come back? Unfortunately, the answer to all three questions has become identical. More food. The perception of value, of *getting your money's worth,* is based on larger and larger portions of food.

The fast-food industry should be credited with the invention of the instantaneously variable portion size. Since the object was to increase the average check, however, the variability only went one way. Up. The industry started with combination meals whose initial appeal was based on ordering convenience and savings. Order a sandwich, fries, and a drink and pay less than ordering the components individually. The combination meals are prominently displayed, so it's easy to make a quick decision to go for the good deal.

After we were all trained to order combination meals, the next great idea was increased sizes. For a nominal increase in price, you could get more fries and a bigger drink. Now, *this* is a great idea. More fries. Yum-yum, fat calories to go in a convenient paper container. Since fries and soda have the highest profit margins, the majority of those 39 cents is pure profit.

Both combination meals and increased sizes are designed to maximize corporate revenue. When a customer arrives at one of the 170,000 fast-food restaurants in the United States,[15] it is imperative that the money spent per customer be maximized. The restaurant's overhead costs are, of course, based on a variety of expenses. Since food costs are low, consistently increasing the average sale through combination meals and increased sizes is a great business decision.

If you examine both the monetary and health costs of these selling techniques, are we, the consumer, making wise decisions while we increase the profits of the fast-food industry?

Figuring the economic cost .s easy. More food for the bargain price of 39 cents. What about the health ramifications? Let's start with the regular order of fries. Anybody out there know how many calories are in a typical order of French fries? How about *440 calories and 19 grams of fat?*

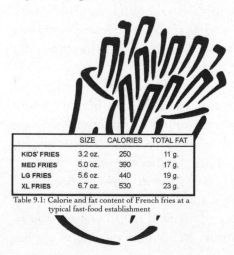

	SIZE	CALORIES	TOTAL FAT
KIDS' FRIES	3.2 oz.	250	11 g.
MED FRIES	5.0 oz.	390	17 g.
LG FRIES	5.6 oz.	440	19 g.
XL FRIES	6.7 oz.	530	23 g.

Table 9.1: Calorie and fat content of French fries at a typical fast-food establishment

And, if you increase the size of those fries? A quick *530 calories and 23 grams of fat.*

What about real soda?

The presence of self-service refills encourages customers to maximize the non-nutritious sugar calories present in soft drinks. Since a higher proportion of males drink sugared soda, the high caloric content of soda is of particular concern for the overweight adolescent male population.

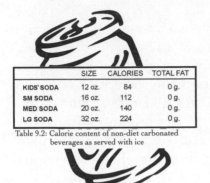

	SIZE	CALORIES	TOTAL FAT
KIDS' SODA	12 oz.	84	0 g.
SM SODA	16 oz.	112	0 g.
MED SODA	20 oz.	140	0 g.
LG SODA	32 oz.	224	0 g.

Table 9.2: Calorie content of non-diet carbonated beverages as served with ice

This information is not presented with the expectation that you'll never eat fast food again, but to emphasize the necessity of making informed choices when ordering fast food. If you're the average woman, 5'4" in height, 164 pounds in weight, and eating 2000 calories per day, an upsized order of fries represents 27 percent of your calories and 35 percent of your fat for the *entire day*. That's *just the fries*. That's before you even touch your sandwich.

In the world of fast food, a child's meal consisting of a cheeseburger, fries, and a diet soda has 577 calories and 26 grams of fat. If she wants a burger . . .

The average woman should be ordering a child's meal, rather than a combination meal.

Remember my own personal favorite and frequently consumed fast-food meal, 1310 calories and 45 grams of fat? Those numbers are based on diet soda. If regular soda is added, the calories increase to 1620, and I'm consuming my entire day's calories at one meal. Spend an extra 39 cents to upsize that meal, and 1720 calories are accompanied by 49 artery-clogging fat grams.

I still eat at the same fast-food restaurant, but now I order a taco salad, and I don't eat the chips. I'm not suffering; I like taco salads. I was just *in the habit* of ordering the chicken combo. I'm changing my habits.

Restaurants

The trend toward increased portion sizes is everywhere. If you sell bagels, make your bagels bigger. How much bigger? If you check a calorie guide, a bagel is listed as having 80 calories. But that's a one-ounce bagel, and the average bagel may weigh three, four, or even five ounces. The bagel purchased from my favorite bagel store weighed three and a half ounces. That's about 280 calories, and that's before you put anything on it. The problem with consistently eating that size bagel is that your stomach begins to think that three and a half ounces of bagel, plus cream cheese, is a normal portion.

If you order lunch at just about any Chinese restaurant, you'll get about two cups of rice. Two cups of rice must be a serving, right? And a serving of rice has about a hundred calories. Well, you're half right. A serving of rice does have about a hundred calories, but a serving is half a cup. You've just been given four servings of rice. And that's white rice, not fried rice. How many of us are ordering white rice, if fried rice is the same price? And what becomes of proper portions at the ever-popular Chinese buffet?

Buffet-style restaurants present a particularly dangerous eating environment, since studies indicate that the amount of food we consume is related to the number of choices we're offered.[16] Combine a clean-plate mentality with unlimited variety, and most of us are in trouble.

Everybody likes getting something for nothing, so the standard first course in many restaurants arrives in the form of chips and salsa, cheese biscuits, or loaves of bread and butter. Instant alleviation of hunger makes everyone content and more tolerant of any delays in service that may occur due to understaffing or other unavoidable problems. Unfortunately, it's easy to consume enough calories in that first *free* course to constitute dinner, before dinner is even ordered, much less arrives and is eaten. The cost of those chips may not show up on the dinner check, but they do show up when you step on the scales.

It's very difficult to lose weight and keep it off, if you eat most of your meals away from home. If you do eat out, you have to be particularly vigilant. You have to become a high-maintenance eater.

"I'd like the Asian salad. But without the sesame noodles or the almonds, and I'd like the dressing on the side. And could you please add cucumbers and red onion?"

"I'd like the Santa Fe chicken. But I'd like the sauce and the bacon and the cheese on the side. And please make sure the breast is skinned. And I'd like a baked potato instead of fries, and the butter and the sour cream on the side."

In the movie *When Harry Met Sally,* Harry Burns (Billy Crystal) says to Sally Albright (Meg Ryan), "'On the side' is a very big thing with you." High-maintenance eating out is dining with Sally Albright. Everything is always on the side.

What other high-maintenance habits do I practice? I keep a food diary. I have accepted the fact that being a healthy weight is an on-going project, and keeping track of how many calories I consume is an integral part of the process.

My daily food diary is not elegant. It's not being preserved for posterity; it's something I do for myself. I sometimes manage to get several consecutive days in a notebook before I misplace it, but it's just as likely to be written down on a scrap of paper. No matter *where* I write it down, though, it's easier for me to keep my caloric intake consistent and controlled *when* I write it down.

Keeping a food diary gives me just a little extra willpower. That pat on the back I get to give myself at the end of a normal-calorie day provides a surprising amount of motivation. In today's world of readily available information, the presence of nutrition labels, on-line restaurant nutrition guides, and calorie counters makes keeping track of calories quite painless. I usually write down my breakfast, morning snack, and lunch calories after I've had lunch. I decide what I'm having for my afternoon snack and for dinner. I add it all up, and I know how many discretionary calories I'll have left after dinner. Since most of our meal choices involve a fair amount of repetition, keeping a food diary gets easier the longer you do it. Am I a perfect eater? No. Do I have days when I eat more than my daily allotment of calories? Yes. But day in, day out, I pay attention to what goes in my mouth. Not only what I eat, but also how much I eat.

I previously ate lots of high-fat, high-sugar, and highly processed food. Now I eat very little of that. Once I started eating nutritious foods in the proper portions, I decided that many products I previously ate in excess simply weren't worth the calories. The longer I ate correctly, the easier it became to discriminate between foods. And when I eat, I'm a high-maintenance eater.

CHAPTER 10

No One's in the Kitchen with Dinah

Eating correctly involves an ongoing and constant battle against the omnipresent high-fat and high-sugar environment in which we live, and eating out magnifies those difficulties. How did we respond to those difficulties? We started cooking again. We believe there are basic survival skills necessary to win the battle against overweight, and rudimentary cooking skills are high on the survival-skill list. If you'll spend at least some time in the kitchen, you'll be able to have more control of the food you eat. And you'll be able to eat a wider variety of food.

As we have moved further and further away from preparing food at home, we have become fatter and fatter, and the quality of the food that we routinely consume has decreased. It is very difficult to eat well if you rely completely on others to prepare your food.

Why is a eucaloric diet easier to follow than a typical diet? More calories. More food. It's easier to eat sensibly when you're not hungry. How can you maximize your calories? How can you have the most control over what goes in your mouth? Cook.

Order meatloaf at a restaurant, and you'll have no idea about the grade of ground beef used to prepare it. Prepare it yourself, and you can choose extra-lean ground beef. Eat out, and you're going to be frustrated by the lack of healthy choices on the menu. Cook, and every meal can taste good *and* be healthy.

When did I become fat? When did my children become fat? When I quit cooking.

I grew up surrounded by cooks. My grandmother, my mother,

and my aunts cooked. My childhood memories of holidays are filled with the sights and sounds and smells of wonderful food. I had always cooked without much regard to calories or fat content and had battled my weight all my life, but my weight only spiraled completely out of control when I stopped cooking. Is my family different? Not according to the statistics.

Food Away from Home

Food away from home is defined as food that is not purchased at a retail store such as a grocery store or a gas station. Food away from home includes pizza that is delivered to a private home and includes take-out Chinese. The number of meals eaten away from home increased from 16 percent in 1977 to 28 percent in 1995.[17] The calories consumed away from home are also rising. The statistics indicate that meals eaten in all types of restaurants contribute a higher percentage of calories and fat than meals eaten at home.[18]

In the last hundred years, the effort required on the part of the consumer to produce meals has been steadily reduced. Homemade has become a style of food, rather than food made at home. Fried chicken comes in a bucket. Biscuits come in cans. Teaching a child to bake cookies has been reduced to taking a premixed, preformed cookie from a package and placing it on a cookie sheet.

We kept telling people that we were losing weight because we were eating really well. But it was difficult to get anyone to believe us. No one believes that it is possible to prepare meals that are low-calorie and low-fat and are also filling and taste good. It is.

How did we lose so much weight? We started to cook again, but we changed the way we cooked. While Brett was reading medical textbooks, and I was reading diet books, Diane was reading cookbooks. I grew up to be a good cook; Diane grew up to be a great cook. While I write prose, Diane creates recipes. We work really well together in the kitchen. Diane will have a suggestion for a new recipe, and we'll bounce it back and forth refining the basic concept. She'll prepare a sample, and we'll taste it. We make changes until we're happy with the result.

While we altered our recipes and devised new ones to meet the caloric and fat requirements of our new eating regime, we ate really well, so we did not suffer the feelings of deprivation that appeared to inevitably lead to bingeing. Most people who are trying to lose weight are eating *horrid* food. They are amazed to discover they can lose weight while eating reasonable portions of excellent food.

In order to convince someone that it's possible to cook good-tasting food that has a reasonable calorie and fat profile, you first have to convince them that it's possible to cook at all. There are starting to be families that consist of multiple generations of noncooks.

Diane learned to cook because she grew up in a house with a mother who cooked. I baked bread and made pizza dough from scratch, and my mashed potatoes came from potatoes rather than a box. This level of cooking skill is no longer common.

If you don't learn to cook at home, your primary exposure to cooking is probably the Food Network, where culinary school–trained professional chefs are preparing fabulous food with ingredients that you can neither pronounce nor spell and that certainly don't reside in your kitchen cupboards. You're completely intimidated, and you're convinced that cooking is hard. You live in a world filled with prepared-food purveyors who want you to believe that *cooking is hard*.

The recipes in this book are designed to provide calorically acceptable versions of basic recipes that anyone with rudimentary cooking skills can prepare. The recipes are presented as menus, as recipes that "go together" and provide complete meals. Meatloaf, Mashed Potatoes, and Country Green Beans. Honey Mustard Chicken, Orzo Pilaf, and Roasted Asparagus.

We give monthly cooking demonstrations, and one woman who attends them confided that her husband had dubbed the Meatloaf recipe "The Seven-Year Meatloaf." They'd been married seven years, and she'd never cooked a meatloaf. In fact, she rarely cooked at all. Now she's cooked many of the recipes in the book, and she's constantly asking for new recipes. (Recipes from the cooking demonstrations are posted on the caloriequeens.com Web site.)

Diane had to make an alteration in the meal schedule last Monday, so she invented a new chicken dish. Later in the week, someone asked when the recipe would be available. Watching people lose weight eating the food we prepare is wonderful, but knowing you're changing the way they cook is even more rewarding. It demonstrates a commitment to lifestyle changes that will help people maintain their weight loss long-term.

We not only teach people to change the way they cook, we also teach them to change the way they shop. Most of us are in a hurry when we shop. We're tired, we're hungry, and we routinely buy the same brands or what's on sale. Diane and I spent a lot of time in grocery stores. We spent a lot of time standing around reading labels and taking notes.

Nutrition Labels

In 1990, Congress passed the Nutrition Labeling and Education Act (NLEA), which was enacted in 1994. This legislation requires all packaged food to carry a nutrition label. The label includes the number of servings per container, the serving size, the calories per serving, and the calories from total and saturated fat. Additional information about cholesterol, sodium, total carbohydrates, dietary fiber, sugar, and protein is also included. The amounts of the vitamins A and D, and the minerals calcium and iron, are listed.

Figure 10.1 provides a sample food label. Labels contain a great deal of information that can be extremely useful in counting calories and fat grams, or determining other relevant health information about a product.

The mind-set that counting calories is a tedious and difficult process is a remnant from the pre–nutrition label days. The presence of nutrition labels on so many food products makes counting calories relatively painless. But for some reason, counting calories continues to be regarded as an unbearably time-consuming and unpleasant task.

When you're reading a label, you do have to pay attention. The information of a label is based on a serving size. If you eat an entire muffin whose calorie and fat information is based on a serving size of *half* a muffin, you have just eaten *twice* as many calories as you thought. If a product is some type of a mix, the nutritional information may be for the mix alone. It is optional to include the nutritional information of the *as prepared* product.

Diane and I purchased a scone mix that listed its caloric content as 110 calories per scone. But that number was based *only* on the contents of the mix. Add milk, eggs, and 12 table-spoons of butter, and the caloric content of the final product is frighteningly different than the number on the box.

But, for the most part, nutrition labels make counting calories no more complicated than counting fat grams or carbohydrates. And everyone seems quite capable of counting both of these.

Making Good Product Choices

One of the most useful ways to use the information on food labels is to compare similar products. We cook Mexican food, so we stood in the aisle of the grocery store and compared tortillas. In addition to variations from brand to brand, there are size variations within a brand.

Figure 10.1: Standard food label

Nutrition Facts

Serving Size 1/2 cup dry (40g)
Servings Per Container see UPC table

Amount Per Serving

	Cereal Alone	with 1/2 cup Vitamin A&D Fortified Skim Milk
Calories	150	190
Calories from Fat	25	25

	% Daily Value**	
Total Fat 3g*	5%	5%
Saturated Fat 0.5g	2%	2%
Polyunsaturated Fat 1g		
Monounsaturated Fat 1g		
Cholesterol 0mg	0%	0%
Sodium 0mg	0%	3%
Total Carbohydrate 27g	9%	11%
Dietary Fiber 4g	15%	15%
Soluble Fiber 2g		
Insoluble Fiber 2g		
Sugars 1g		
Protein 5g		
Vitamin A	0%	4%
Vitamin C	0%	2%
Calcium	0%	15%
Iron	10%	10%

*Amount in Cereal. One half cup skim milk contributes an additional 40 Calories, 65mg Sodium, 200mg Potassium, 6g Total Carbohydrate (6g Sugars), and 4g Protein.
**Percent Daily Values are based on a 2,000 calorie diet. Your daily values may be higher or lower depending on your calorie needs:

	Calories	2,000	2,500
Total Fat	Less than	65g	80g
Sat. Fat	Less than	20g	25g
Cholesterol	Less than	300mg	300mg
Sodium	Less than	2,400mg	2,400mg
Total Carbohydrate		300g	375g
Dietary Fiber		25g	30g

Calories per gram:
Fat 9 • Carbohydrate 4 • Protein 4

Now, a tortilla is basically a neutral starch used to wrap around other food. Why not choose the tortilla with the lowest number of calories and the least amount of fat? Is it a big deal? Remember the discussions about portion sizes?

We've trained ourselves to routinely consume portions that are too large. We need to learn to eat smaller portions. If two tacos is a normal serving of tacos, reducing the calories in the tacos by using a fajita-sized tortilla instead of a taco-sized tortilla reduces the calories in the tortillas by 140 calories and 8 grams of fat.

Table 10.2: Calorie and fat content of tortillas

	Calories	Fat Grams
Kroger, fajita-sized tortilla	80	0.5
Kroger, taco-sized tortilla	150	4.0
Kroger, burrito-sized tortilla	220	5.0
Old El Paso, tortilla	80	2.25
Aztec, tortilla	130	2.5
Mission, burrito-sized tortilla	220	5.0

But it also takes less meat and cheese to fill the smaller tortilla. Perhaps rather than three ounces of meat per taco, you use two ounces of meat, and one ounce of cheese instead of two. That saves approximately 100 calories and 3 grams of fat in meat, and 110 calories and 9 grams of fat in cheese. Suddenly there's a total difference of 350 calories and 20 grams of fat. If you eat tacos twice a month for a year, that savings is equal to the calories in about two pounds of body fat.

A main course for dinner that consists of two tortillas, four ounces of meat, one ounce of cheese, lettuce, and tomato equals 470 calories and 15 grams of fat. This meal meets the government recommendations of no more than 30 percent of calories from fat. Add a salad with low-fat dressing, or full-fat dressing on the side, and you have a great dinner that doesn't make you feel deprived before you even sit down.

The most important fact is that eating smaller tacos is a better choice than not eating tacos at all. The fastest way to start feeling deprived is to start treating any food as forbidden or illegal. We made adjustments in our recipes, and our portion sizes, so we could eat everything. We didn't feel deprived, so we didn't binge. We lost the weight we wanted to lose, and we have kept the weight off.

Similar variations exist in every other product. Bread varies from 40 calories and .25 grams of fat per slice for light to 150 calories and 2 grams of fat per slice for regular. Again, is it a big deal? Over a lifetime of bread consumption, the answer is clearly yes.

By paying a little more attention to the brands you purchase, it's possible to make a significant difference in your overall calorie and fat consumption. Will making these types of changes cause you to lose ten pounds in forty-eight hours or nine inches off your waist in thirty days? No, but it may cause you to lose five or ten pounds in a year. And it will represent the loss of fat, not water. And that weight is more likely to stay lost, rather than return with friends.

Low-Fat Versus Fat-Free

There are presently thousands of food items that are available in regular, low-fat, and fat-free versions. We substitute reduced-calorie products, *if we think they're an acceptable substitute for the real thing*. Otherwise, we adjust the amount we use. Eliminating any food group stokes up the deprivation/binge-eating demons, so we haven't eliminated anything from our diet.

There are reports that, as a result of reduced-fat choices, Americans have decreased the percentage of fat in our diets. But we are not losing weight. We are gaining weight, because we've increased our daily caloric intake. *Fat-free food is not calorie-free food.*

The fat that is eliminated from these products is often replaced with sugar. Just because a bag contains fat-free chips doesn't mean that you can eat the entire bag. The body can and does convert excess calories from fat-free food into excess body fat.

EXTRA-LEAN BEEF

One major change in our cooking is utilizing the low-fat meat products that are becoming readily available. These products allow traditional *home-cooked* meals to be prepared without sacrificing flavor to achieve reduced calorie and fat content. We use 96 percent extra-lean ground beef in all our recipes.

If you decide after reading this book to make one single change in your life and forget everything else, this is the change to make.

**Never, ever use anything but 96 percent
extra-lean ground beef.**

Since ground beef is the basis of so many standard family recipes, the savings in calories achieved by using the leaner beef makes a tremendous difference in daily calorie consumption.

Why Does It Make So Much Difference?
The problem with ground beef is the information printed on the label. Ground beef is generally labeled "85/15," 85 percent lean and 15 percent fat, or "90/10," 90 percent lean and 10 percent fat. The price of the ground beef naturally increases as the percent of fat on the label decreases. How many of us are willing to spend the money on 96/4, extra-lean ground beef, when it's so much more expensive than 85/15 beef? After all, 85/15 is only 15 percent fat, right? That doesn't sound too bad.

Unfortunately, 85/15 ground beef is 15 percent fat *by weight*, which is fairly useless information because a high percentage of the weight in ground beef is water weight that has no calories. It doesn't matter how much fat *physically* weighs—a three-ounce cupcake weighs less than an eight-ounce glass of water, but that doesn't mean you'll consume fewer calories by eating the cupcake than by drinking the water.

The 85 percent lean, 15 percent fat information is usually in large, easily read type. If you look at the information on the nutrition label, however, you can determine that a four-ounce serving of 85/15 ground beef contains 240 calories and that 150 of those calories come from fat. Let's do a little math.

$$150 \div 240 = .625$$

Multiply by 100 to get the percentage.

$$.625 \times 100 = 62.5\%$$

The 85/15 ground beef may be 15 percent fat *by weight*, but it's 62.5 percent fat *by calories*. Let's repeat that in large letters just in case you weren't paying enough attention.

62.5 percent of the calories in 85/15 ground beef come from fat!

Table 10.3 shows the difference between percent fat by weight and percent fat by calories. It's an ugly surprise to discover that the

Table 10.3: Percent fat in ground beef based on caloric content

Serving size 4 ounces					
% Lean by weight	% Fat by weight	Calories (total)	Calories (from fat)	% Lean by calories	% Fat by calories
80	20	290	200	31	69
85	15	240	150	38	62
90	10	190	90	53	47
96	04	130	25	81	19

90/10 ground beef you naturally assumed was 10 percent fat by calories is actually 47 percent fat by calories.

Why is ground beef responsible for such a high percentage of the saturated fat in our diet? We're buying 85/15 or 90/10 ground beef and feeling virtuous, because we don't understand that the label on the ground beef isn't telling us what we think it is. *Even the leanest grade of ground beef still gets 19 percent of its calories from fat.*

If I'm on a typical, temporary diet, I could simply not eat beef while I'm trying to lose weight. But I'm not on a temporary diet, I'm making permanent changes in my eating habits. I'm *not* willing to give up beef forever. I *am* willing to pay for the leanest beef product available. I *am* willing to use ground beef in dishes that also contain vegetables and starches. These recipes allow the meat portion of the dish to be reduced to a calorically acceptable level without giving up the taste of beef that we want.

Extra-lean ground beef is more expensive, but other grades of beef simply contain too many calories and too much fat to be an option for me. It is possible to produce reasonable servings that contain acceptable calories and fat by using extra-lean ground beef.

LEAN PORK

We eat lots of pork; we just choose the leanest cuts available—the center-cut pork loin or the pork tenderloin. Since the calorie and fat content varies greatly between brands, it is necessary to purchase pork that carries a nutrition label. We try to buy pork with 120–140 calories and 3–4.5 grams of fat in a four-ounce portion. This pork compares favorably to chicken in calories, with only a slightly higher fat content.

The most critical factor in preparing pork that tastes good is the cooking time. Concern about trichinosis and other diseases caused by worm organisms created a generation of cooks who overcooked pork with a vengeance. When pork was cooked to an internal temperature of 170°F, it resembled shoe leather.

It is now recognized that worm organisms are killed at an internal temperature of 137°F, and modern recommendations for cooking pork generally list 140°F as the safe temperature. Buy a meat thermometer and give pork a chance. You'll be pleasantly surprised.

The use of lean beef and lean pork enables us to significantly lower the calories in our recipes. The more recipes we altered, the easier it was to continue dieting successfully. These changes are not temporary changes. These are long-term changes to the recipes that compose our standard daily fare, our diet.

MILK/DAIRY PRODUCTS

I drink milk and eat yogurt so I won't have osteoporosis when I'm an old lady (and because I like them). I "trained" myself to eat and drink the lower-fat versions of these products.

There are a variety of food items whose variation in calories is the result of using higher- or lower-fat milk products. There are reduced-calorie sour cream, cottage cheese, cream cheese, and yogurt, as well as fat-free versions of the same products. Using the lower-fat milk products can make a significant difference in the calorie and fat content of a recipe.

I eat the reduced-fat versions of these products. I don't use the fat-free versions; I don't like the taste. But you should try them for yourself; you may disagree with me.

The milk label is similar to the ground beef label. Milk is another product whose label lists calories by weight. Table 10.4 shows the percentage of calories from fat in the various dairy products.

Table 10.4: Percent fat in dairy products based on caloric content

	Calories		Calories
Skim milk	80/cup	Reduced-fat cream cheese	60/ounce
1% Milk	130/cup	Regular cream cheese	80/ounce
2% Milk	140/cup	Low-fat sour cream	324/cup
3.5% Milk	160/cup	Regular sour cream	492/cup
Half & Half	317/cup	Low-fat cottage cheese	160/cup
Medium cream	608/cup	Reduced-fat cottage cheese	200/cup
Heavy cream	792/cup	Regular cottage cheese	240/cup

CHEESE AS A CONDIMENT

Perhaps no other single item in our diet was altered more than our consumption of cheese. Cheese is one of my favorite foods, and I always purchased it in those handy eight-ounce packages. It never occurred to me that a casserole should be covered by anything less than an entire package.

Even if we use lower-fat milk products, most of us manage to ignore the fact that most cheeses are "full-fat" dairy products. Cheese is a combination food; it contains both protein and fat. But, at 110 calories and 9 grams of fat per ounce, the typical cheese is fairly comparable to any of the fats listed in Table 10.5. Cheese is an energy-dense food, and it's possible to add a tremendous number of calories and fat grams very quickly with cheese.

Have we quit using cheese? No. We're just much more careful about the amount we consume. In my previous life, an 8-ounce package was a reasonable portion of cheese. Today, my refrigerator contains cheese "pats," individually wrapped three-quarter-ounce packages that go nicely with an apple as a midmorning snack for 160 calories and 7 grams of fat.

We also use part-skim mozzarella and part-skim ricotta. If a recipe calls for cheese, and mozzarella will give the right taste, it's a better calorie and fat choice than cheddar. Using sharp cheddar rather than mild or medium cheddar helps add the desired flavor without using as much cheese.

FAT

No discussion of changes in diet can be complete without discussing fat. The fat category encompasses oil, butter, and mayonnaise. The table below lists calories and fat grams for common fats.

Table 10.5: Calorie and fat content of common fats

	Calories	Fat grams
Butter, 1 tablespoon	100	11
Margarine, 1 tablespoon	100	11
Vegetable oil, 1 tablespoon	120	14
Mayonnaise, 1 tablespoon	100	11
Lard, 1 tablespoon	115	13

Cheese, fats, chocolate, and nuts are all considered energy-dense foods, because the calorie to weight ratio is so high. It is, therefore, possible to consume a massive number of calories without any satiation of hunger due to the density of calories in these foods.

Food Claims

Food labels help make eating correctly much easier. They provide a wealth of information about our food choices. They make paying attention to the food we eat much easier, but deciding whether you're eating correctly can still be a challenge. Sometimes it's necessary to understand exactly what standard has been set for a particular definition. If a label advertises a food as being fat-free, cholesterol-free, low-sodium, or high-fiber, the food must meet well-defined criteria.

Low-fat—contains less than 3 grams of fat per serving.
Fat-free—contains less than a half a gram of fat per serving.
Calorie-free—contains 4 or fewer calories per serving.
Sugar-free—contains less than half a gram of sugar per serving.
Cholesterol-free—contains less than two milligrams of cholesterol per serving.

Carbohydrate-free—contains less than half a gram of carbohydrates per serving.
Fiber-free—contains less than half a gram of fiber per serving.
Protein-free—contains less than half a gram of protein per serving.

If a food product claims to be low in some nutrient, or reduced, it must be in reference to a similar product. By definition, a reduced-fat product must have 25 percent less fat than the comparable full-fat product. So a reduced-fat cookie will have at least 25 percent less fat than the comparable regular cookie, but that doesn't qualify the cookie as low-fat unless it also has less than 3 grams of fat per serving.

A low-sodium product must have less than 140 milligrams of sodium per serving; a very-low-sodium product must have less than 35 milligrams of sodium per serving. This designation only applies to products that are not naturally low in sodium. Chicken broth is available as regular, low-sodium, and very-low-sodium. Frozen or fresh corn is naturally low in sodium, so it is not labeled low- or very-low-sodium. In order to make claims regarding low or reduced products, something must have been done to that product to make it that way.

Similarly, if a label states that a product is fortified or enriched, it must have at least 10 percent more of the daily recommended value of protein, vitamins, minerals, dietary fiber, or potassium than some reference product. A good source must have 10–19 percent more, while a high source must have at least 20 percent more of the specific nutrient than the reference product.

Things are less clear when the adjective used is "light" or "lite." Technically, a "light" product indicates that a product which normally derives more than 50 percent of its calories from fat has reduced its calories by at least 50 percent. Butter is a good example of this situation. Butter has 100 calories and 11 grams of fat per tablespoon, and it derives essentially all its calories from fat. Light butter has 50 calories and 6 grams of fat in a tablespoon.

However, regular olive oil and light olive oil both have 120 calories and 14 grams of fat per tablespoon. Why? In this example, the "light" in the product description refers to the strength of the olive flavor in the oil. Light brown sugar refers to the color and molasses content of the brown sugar.

If you've never paid any attention to food labels, you'll be surprised how much information they provide, and how much easier they make it to keep track of your calories.

CHAPTER II

Sensible Goals

When I talk to people about weight loss, I'm in a unique position. Whether I'm talking to someone who's morbidly obese or someone who wants to lose ten pounds, I understand where both of them are coming from. I know that the woman who needs to lose a hundred pounds is *aching* to smack the skinny broad who's whining about needing to lose ten pounds squarely on her size 8 butt. I now realize that the skinny broad (who is actually a very nice woman who spends an hour every day running on a treadmill) is not technically skinny, and she's tired of being treated like it's *easy* for her to be a reasonable weight. And she'd *really* like to weigh about ten pounds less than she does, and she's *not* whining.

Diane and I work with a registered dietician. She's a very nice woman who has never had a weight problem. When she talks to people who are morbidly obese about making changes in their lives, she knows where they need *to be*, but it's impossible for her to understand where they *are*. She's never been there. When we talk to people about making changes, we know *exactly* what we're asking. But we can also assure them that change is possible.

In order to lose weight, we have to decide to do something tomorrow that is different than what we've done today. Because what we've done today is keeping us heavier than we would like to be.

There are three common motivations for us to make changes in our lives in order to lose weight: appearance, current health, and future health. When concern about appearance is the major motivation, there are two key measurements of success (or failure): the number on the scales and the size on the garment tags.

Scales

Take a look at my birthday and an astrological chart, and you'll discover I'm a Libra. That has always seemed depressingly appropriate; I had certainly spent most of my life obsessed with scales. I *always* weighed myself at least once a day. If I was dieting and having a bad day, I weighed myself multiple times. The *worse* I was, the more necessary the weigh-ins, as if weighing myself would provide tangible proof of the need for deprivation, and somehow stop the bingeing. If I was having a *good* day or *several* good days, I could be satisfied with a once-a-day weigh-in, but I expected instant response from the scales to prove that the sacrifices associated with dieting were being appropriately rewarded.

At lower weights, there is great power in a change in the tens column of one's weight. When I was in high school, I weighed between 120 and 129 pounds. I never seemed to be able to get below 120, but whenever I got to 129 pounds, I managed to muster the willpower to diet back down to 120. For me, the mental difference between 129 and 130 always seemed more significant than the physical difference between 120 and 129.

As I got older, my weight gradually increased. Each decade appeared to correlate with the next fifty-pound increment on the scales. I had spent my thirties struggling between 150 pounds and 200 pounds. During my forties, the battle had moved to the 200- and 250-pounds level, and the last few years I had remained at the upper end of that range. Whenever my weight approached 250 pounds, I'd diet long enough to lose ten or twenty pounds. In the summer of 2000, I had reason to be nervous; I was getting close to the next decade.

Did this pattern indicate I was looking at weighing 500 pounds in my eighties? Even at that weight, I still wouldn't be in the running for the Guinness World Record for fatness, but, quite frankly, that had never been one of my life's goals.

When Diane and I started changing our daily fare, the scales went to live in the garage. I didn't weigh myself for six months.

Diane didn't weigh herself for a year. We both had so much weight to lose that whether we lost one pound or three pounds each week didn't really matter. We just needed to keep eating 1600 calories day after day. We knew if we ate correctly, the weight would come off. It didn't matter how long it took.

Where are the scales today? They're in the garage. They were in the laundry room, but I've finally admitted to myself that daily or weekly weigh-ins make it harder for me to eat properly.

When I'm faithfully keeping my food diary and eating well, I don't *need* to get on the scales. It's only when I'm struggling that I feel the need to weigh myself. It is easier for me to eat consistently when I don't have easy access to a set of scales.

Garment Tags

Clothing size can also influence our eating decisions, but clothing size is more complicated than the weight shown on a set of scales. Scales are empirical devices that measure the effect of gravity on our earthbound bodies. The size displayed on a clothing tag *can* and *is* being manipulated.

In the 1970s, there was a voluntary effort by manufacturers to standardize women's sizes. The size 8 established by the PS 42–70 standard fit dimensions of 33"-24"-35". The increasing size of today's population has made those standard fit dimensions completely outdated. A survey of sixteen of today's women's apparel manufacturers indicated that the dimensions of today's size eight are 36"-27"-37½", an increase of 3" in the bust, 3" in the waist, and 2½" in the hips over the 1970 standard. Yesterday's size 8 is today's size 4. Sizes 0 and 2 were created so that clothing with larger dimensions could still have acceptable numbers on the labels.

Who among us has not purchased a garment that was clearly larger than expected for the size on the tag? When I was wearing a size 14, I tried on a blouse. It was unexpectedly large. I tried the size 12. I tried the size 10. Finally, the size 8 fit. I bought the blouse.

A tape measure would surely have demonstrated that the dimensions of that blouse were identical to another manufacturer's size 14, but I couldn't help being seduced by the size 8 on the label. Even though I knew the size on the tag wasn't accurate, I still bought the blouse. I stood in the store and discussed all of this with Diane, but *I still bought the blouse*!

Why are manufacturers using "vanity" sizing? It works.

Changing Goals

Why *should* we be concerned if we're overweight or obese? Our health. If you're presently overweight or obese, and you're still healthy, it's probably time to move the "future health" motivation to the top of the list.

There's a frightening list of health risks associated with being overweight and obese, and both the degree of overweight and the distribution of body fat affect the risk of developing the following problems:[19]

- Insulin resistance, type 2 diabetes
- Hyperlipidemia
- Hypertension
- Coronary heart disease
- Stroke
- Some types of cancer
- Gastroesophageal reflux disease
- Gallstones, gallbladder disease
- Gout
- Nonalcoholic fatty liver disease
- Pregnancy complications
- Menstrual irregularities
- Bladder control problems, stress incontinence
- Osteoarthritis
- Obstructive sleep apnea, respiratory problems
- Infertility
- Psychological disorders

If you presently have obesity-related health problems, it's important to remember that even modest weight losses of 5–10 percent have been shown to be beneficial in improving obesity-related health problems.

The Last Ten Pounds

What if you just want to lose ten pounds? Does Eucalorics have anything to offer you?

We've been cooking for our church's accountant for the last three years. She came downstairs one day and asked if we only prepared food for people who needed to lose *lots* of weight. She wanted to lose fifteen or twenty pounds, but she was primarily interested in a healthy dinner that someone else cooked. We started preparing her dinner, and she gradually lost the weight she wanted to lose. When I asked her about her experience, this is what she said:

"Many years—many diets. Put it on. Take it off. I always looked forward to the 'end of a diet' so I could return to my old way of eating. After Eucalorics I don't want to go back. I like this food better! And I'll never have to 'diet' again!"

Losing ten pounds with Eucalorics uses exactly the same approach as losing a hundred pounds. But when you're at a significantly lower starting weight, the math looks different. Remember the extra calories calculation in chapter 9? When I weighed 247 pounds, I was averaging almost 3000 calories a day to maintain that weight. When I started eating the 1600 calories a day that maintains 135 pounds, I had a calorie deficit of approximately 1400 calories per day. Since there are 3500 calories in a pound, the first pound was lost in two and a half days.

$$\frac{3500 \text{ calories/pound}}{1400 \text{ calories/day}} = 2\frac{1}{2} \text{ days/pound}$$

What happens to the numbers if you want to lose ten pounds? If you weigh 135 pounds, and you want to weigh 125 pounds, what do the numbers look like?

135 pounds × 12 calories/pound = 1620 calories
125 pounds × 12 calories/pound = 1500 calories
1620 calories − 1,500 calories = 120 calories

The difference between weighing 135 pounds and weighing 125 pounds is only 120 calories a day!

Most people's instinctive response to this little bit of information is disbelief. It just doesn't seem possible that so few calories could make that much difference. But they do.

Want more proof? I can get the same answer with a slightly different calculation. Remember the 12 calories per pound calculation? Apply the math to ten pounds, and look where you end up.

$$10 \text{ pounds} \times 12 \text{ calories/pound} = 120 \text{ calories}$$

Why is it so hard to lose the last ten pounds?

There's very little difference in daily caloric intake between ten-pound intervals of weight. Since there are 3500 calories in a pound, you have to wait until those 120 calories a day add up to 3500 calories to lose just one pound.

$$\frac{3500 \text{ calories/pound}}{120 \text{ calories/day}} = 29 \text{ days/pound}$$

$$10 \text{ pounds} \times 29 \text{ days/pound} = 290 \text{ days}$$

$$\frac{290 \text{ days}}{30 \text{ days/month}} = 9.67 \text{ months}$$

It will take almost ten months to lose those ten pounds. Remember the chocolate coins at the bank, mints by the restaurant cashier, and toffees at the dry cleaners? Or "cleaning" your children's plates of those few extra bites before they go in the dishwasher? Or that extra handful of chips?

It's really easy to eat an extra 120 calories a day.

How much food is 120 calories? It's approximately . . .

- 28 peanuts
- 1½-ounce roll
- 8-ounce apple
- 1 cup 2% milk
- 30 Jelly Bellies or 30 M&M's
- 1½ ounces cheese
- 8 cups 94% fat-free popcorn

Most people who want to lose "just a few pounds" don't realize how little difference there is between the calories that support what they presently weigh and the calories that support what they want to weigh. When I talk to people about choosing a goal weight, I ask them to begin by taking a good look at what they *think* they want to weigh.

If you're within ten pounds of being happy with what you weigh, take a moment to consider how extremely lucky that makes you. If you're maintaining your present weight relatively easily, maybe you should quit being so hard on yourself and give some serious thought to being happy with your present weight.

If you really want to weigh ten pounds less, take the time to figure out where those extra 120 calories a day are coming from. Make some minor adjustments in your diet and get on with your life. Eliminate 120 calories a day, quit obsessing about your weight, and ten months from now you'll be ten pounds lighter.

Or go to the gym four days a week and burn 300 calories.

Which should you choose?

Go to the gym.

What should we be doing to improve our health besides improve our diets? We need to be getting some exercise. Get off the couch, turn off the TV, and get your body moving.

CHAPTER 12

The Evil Empire of Exercise

In June of 2000, we were primarily interested in losing weight. Ultimately, however, our goals shifted. We became less interested in the final number on the scales and became more interested in our overall health. Despite disagreement on the exact relationship between diet and exercise, there's little disagreement among health professionals that moderate physical activity is an important component of a healthy lifestyle.

Why do the government recommendations for health include recommendations for physical activity?

Regular physical activity is beneficial to maintaining a normal weight, but its benefits extend far beyond weight control. Regular exercise improves our blood lipid profile. It lowers our blood cholesterol, removes cholesterol deposits from the walls of blood vessels, and reduces our risk from heart attack and stroke. Regular exercise improves our endurance by improving the condition of our muscles, including our heart. Exercise helps us stay active as we age, by maintaining joint flexibility and by preserving bone mass that prevents osteoporosis.

Exercise facilitates the loss of body fat by increasing energy expenditure and metabolism, and by protecting your lean body mass.

Why should you care about your muscle mass? Our muscle cells are the most metabolically active tissue in the body; our lean muscle mass burns calories. The better your body's ratio of lean muscle to fat, the more calories your body burns, whether you're walking on a treadmill or sitting on a sofa. If you reduce your lean muscle mass, you decrease your body's ability to metabolize calories.

What about fat? Fat is essentially inert. Fat spends its days doing *nothing*.

Fat cells are couch potatoes at the molecular level!

Remember the 12 calories per pound formula? That formula was based on an inactive person. If you exercise while you're losing weight, you not only lose weight more quickly, you also help maintain your muscle mass. Once you get to your goal weight, you'll be able to eat more while maintaining your weight. You'll be burning calories while exercising, and your body will have more metabolically active muscle tissue.

If you are female, you have a naturally higher percentage of body fat and less muscle mass. Since women are normally shorter and smaller-framed, it also takes fewer calories to maintain a normal weight. Making exercise part of your daily life allows you to eat a few more discretionary calories and still stay within the normal weight range.

Life used to provide plenty of exercise, but modern life provides very little. Food is more readily available, and most of us no longer lead lives that require the level of caloric intake that we consume. A few hundred years ago, we were a society of farmers and laborers whose day-to-day survival depended on hard physical labor. Today, we are a nation of sedentary office workers who use telephones, computers, and automobiles to conduct our business. Women no longer scrub clothes down by the riverside and hang them outside to dry. Chicken dinner doesn't start with a chicken pecking seeds in the backyard, but with chicken fried at the fast-food restaurant.

Since our jobs no longer require physical labor, exercise must be incorporated into our *leisure-time* schedules. However, recent government statistics indicate that 25 percent of adults engage in *no* physical activity. None. Nada. Zip. And less than half of us presently meet the government recommendations of regular moderate physical activity for at least 30 minutes per day.[20]

I'd been a lifetime member of the Coach Potato Hall of Fame, and I went kicking and screaming into a pair of gym shoes. I could spell "exercise," but I didn't like to get that close to it. And as far as I was concerned, sweat was what formed on the outside of a wineglass on a warm day.

For the first eight weeks, all we did was diet. For those fifty-six days, the most important thing was staying on the diet. After eight weeks we started exercising. We started by walking around the neighborhood. The first few weeks were tremendously pitiful. I whined while I walked, and my thigh muscles twitched in horrified protest at the scorching one-mile-per-hour pace. We walked four to five times a week and gradually (*very* gradually) increased the pace.

When the weather started to get bad, we headed to the local mall. The majority of the morning walking crowd consisted of slender "senior" citizens who zipped merrily around us. (Nothing more humiliating than being lapped by people on Medicare.) It was, however, very convincing evidence that exercise is good for you.

At the end of a year, we decided to join a gym. By the time this book goes to print, Diane and I will have belonged to the Lexington Athletic Club for four years. And I do more than simply belong. When I walk through the door, people recognize me. In the locker room, I know names.

It's a really nice athletic club filled with good equipment, a friendly staff, and a surprising number of people who claim they actually enjoy being there! (These people were evidently paying attention when they started passing out the "likes to exercise" genes. I was in the used bookstore perusing trashy romance novels and didn't hear the announcement.)

I'm living proof that it's possible to exercise without loving it. You don't even have to like it very much. You *do* need to feel guilty if you don't do it. It needs to be like brushing your teeth, washing the makeup off your face at night, and wearing clean underwear every morning. It needs to be on the list of things you do. Period.

Unfortunately, the heavier we are, the more difficult exercise may be. The less we exercise, the less muscle we maintain, and a cycle of weight gain accompanied by less and less activity can develop.

The most important thing is to do something. Do as much as you can, but be sensible. Don't overdo. It's far more important to do a little each day, day after day, than to do too much on any one day. You'll get hurt and quit. The remarkable thing is that if you continue to do a little each day, then a little more each day, you suddenly discover you can do more than you ever thought possible.

> If you have significant health problems associated with being overweight, your primary care physician should make recommendations before you begin any exercise regimen.

Exercising needs to be as much a habit as eating a proper diet. Exercise needs to be part of a permanent change in your lifestyle. The rewards can be amazing. It is truly remarkable that my body could forgive the years of abuse to which it had been subjected. I'd been morbidly obese for a decade, but my body didn't hold it against me.

Brett and I went to Hilton Head Island, and we rode a tandem bicycle all over the island. Diane and I went to New York City, and walked for blocks. We walked for hours, when we previously couldn't have walked for more than a few minutes.

Am I thin? No. But I'm in the best physical shape of my life.

Fit Versus Fat

There are numerous medical professionals who argue against the focus on weight. They insist that fitness, not fatness, is the crucial element in determining health. And even if overweight is identified as a health risk for certain diseases, is the overweight significant in an individual with no risk factors?

The situation is complicated, because definitive correlations between weight and health are impossible to empirically establish. While it is generally agreed that morbid obesity is unhealthy, it is not clear how much excess weight makes health risks become health problems.

There are studies indicating that overweight individuals who exercise may be healthier than individuals of normal weight who do not exercise, but what about people who are not simply overweight but are obese or morbidly obese? The heavier we become, the less likely it is that we exercise. Although it is theoretically possible for people to be fit and fat, it is not the norm.

When I weighed 247 pounds, I was not fit. And there was no way I was going to become fit at that weight. In order to be able to do the physical activities that would help me become fit, I first had to lose weight.

So, you're learning new proper eating habits. You're losing weight. You're exercising. Do you feel good about yourself? You should.

If you can only be happy when you get thin thighs, you may be doomed to disappointment. There are certain unpleasant truths that need to be addressed when discussing exercise and weight loss. As discussed earlier, losing weight does not change the basic shape of our bodies; it just makes the basic shape smaller. A great deal of our body habitus is genetically ordained.

There have been innumerable people who have become rich selling potions, creams, and a wide variety of machines that promise to remove fat from a specific area of the body. But fat is systemic. This means that the charming bulges on the outside of your thighs, my thighs, and everyone else's thighs is fat that just happens to be stored on the outside of the thighs. It is visiting your thighs, but it is not *thigh* fat. It is body fat. It is fat that is being stored by the body to provide energy when the next great famine or diet begins. The only way to lose fat from your thighs is to lose fat from your entire body. And even after you lose a great deal of weight, you may still have thigh bulges.

In order to have washboard abs or a buff butt or not have old-lady, batwing arms, first you have to lose the excess body fat. *After* you've lost the excess body fat, you have to tone specific muscle groups to produce the sculptured musculature that all endorsers of diet products seem to have magically obtained without diet or exercise.

If Hollywood is to provide our standard for physical beauty, we need to be objective in our analysis of that standard. Based on the body mass index charts, most of the female Hollywood population is underweight. In addition to nonstandard heights and weights, the number of Hollywood physiques that owe a great deal to multi-hour-per-day workouts is considerable. For each genetically blessed individual, there is another rigidly disciplined personality who watches every calorie and spends hours with a personal trainer.

Most women who are underweight are not particularly well endowed. I would have to weigh less than 101 pounds to be underweight; at that weight, my chest would probably be concave. Based on this personal observation, the underweight Hollywood population is either genetically or surgically blessed. And, in addition to breast implants, surgeons can change noses, chins, cheekbones, and a myriad of other flaws. How much of what we compare ourselves to is a surgical illusion assisted by makeup, hair extensions, and designer clothing?

So, even though I've lost more than a hundred pounds, I still have to periodically remind myself that I'm not *ever* going to look like Catherine Zeta-Jones (I'm too short).

But losing weight and exercising has given me things far more valuable. It's given me the ability to climb flights of stairs without gasping for breath. It's given me the energy to walk beside my husband without needing him to slow down. It's given me hope for a longer, healthier life.

It's even given me *thinner* thighs.

Sharing a Miracle

Losing a hundred pounds was the answer to more than one desperate prayer for help. But it was, quite frankly, an unexpected answer. Losing twenty pounds would have been a *satisfactory* answer. Losing fifty pounds would have been a *great* answer. Losing a hundred pounds? *That was a miracle.*

In the summer of 2001, we had been dieting for a year. We were incorporating the theories of Eucalorics into our lives. We were dieting and losing weight; we had started working on this book. Brett was reading, I was writing, and Diane was cooking.

Our lives changed when a close friend, David, had symptoms of a stroke. Medically, it was classified as a TIA, a transient ischemic attack, since the symptoms all resolved within twenty-four hours. But his personal physician issued another in a long line of warnings. David had multiple health problems: high cholesterol, high blood pressure, and type 2 diabetes, all aggravated by excess weight. The TIA was a warning. If David did not change his eating habits and lifestyle, he was clearly at risk for a more serious stroke that might either disable him or kill him. His wife, Jackie, left the doctor's office and began to pray for help.

When Brett told Diane and me about David's TIA, we offered to begin cooking dinner for them. Our ideas and recipes were working well for us; perhaps they would also work for David. Initially, David and Jackie were concerned that our cooking for them would be too much work. After some discussion, we agreed that we would try it. If it became too much trouble, we would tell them.

Every Monday through Friday, David and Jackie would come to our house and pick up dinner. It was weighed and measured and packed in plastic containers. Every night we exchanged empty containers for filled containers, and David and Jackie headed home with the first "Eucalorics-To-Go." We began to cook for David and Jackie in July 2001, and they gradually began to lose weight.

Jackie didn't tell us until much later about her prayers. We, who had received an answer to our own prayers, had become the answer to someone else's prayers. We were given a chance to share our miracle.

David is now maintaining a seventy-pound weight loss. His blood lipid profile is better; his cholesterol and triglycerides have improved. Most importantly, he has not had another TIA, or a more serious stroke. Jackie has lost forty pounds. Both of them would like to lose a few more pounds, but they're healthier, and they've made lifestyle changes that are helping them maintain their weight loss.

The Temple Reconstruction Project

We sing in our church choir, and choir members, who had been watching our family lose weight, were now watching David and Jackie lose weight as well. People started to ask, "Are you going to start cooking for anybody else?" In January 2002, our church gave us permission to use their commercial kitchen. We recruited a small group and started the Temple Reconstruction Project.

> **Do you not know that your body is a temple of the**
> **Holy Spirit, who is in you, whom you have received from God?**
> **You are not your own.**
> —1 Corinthians 6:19

Our little group had chef surprise every night, while we experimented with techniques and recipes. We planned to cook for twelve weeks. Twelve weeks was followed by another twelve weeks. Then another. We ended up cooking for our dieters for a year and a half. People came to the basement of the First United Methodist Church and picked up dinner four nights a week. Dinner that was weighed and measured and labeled.

The wife of one of our ministers participated in our group, and he had the following observations to make.

> I remember thinking, "Does some new diet really qualify as a ministry?" The experiences that would soon follow convinced me that what Diane and Jackie have to offer really is life changing.
>
> My wife had been struggling for more than ten years, since the birth of our last child, with being overweight. She was unhappy and self-conscious about her weight. I showed her the article about the Temple Reconstruction Project and suggested that she become one of the volunteers.
>
> She got involved, and over the next eighteen months, lost sixty-five pounds. The number of pounds tells only a small part of the story. Her success was noticed and frequently complimented by our friends. I was happy to support her progress by agreeing to frequent replacements in her wardrobe, as sizes got smaller. The results continue. She is obviously happier, far more confident, and full of energy. I am very proud of her.
>
> The change is more than just a temporary diet plan for losing weight, it is a lifestyle change that is reasonable enough to stay committed to. The result is that her weight loss is sustained and we are all eating healthier.

It's wonderful to have the chance to not only change your own life, but also to help change other people's lives. If you talk to Diane about helping change someone's life, she'll always talk about Katie.

Katie was the youngest participant in the Temple Reconstruction Project. She was a normal-weight two-year-old with two morbidly obese parents, so the statistics for her future weight didn't look good. Parental obesity more than doubles the risk for adult obesity for both obese and non-obese children.[21]

While her parents were trying to learn new eating habits, Katie started life with good eating habits. She eats carrots and broccoli and asparagus. She eats chicken and meatloaf and pork roast. She got half of an adult portion, and she learned to eat food the average two-year-old didn't, because this was the food she was given. Katie thought fast food came from the basement at the First United Methodist Church.

How are Katie's parents doing? Her dad's lost about a hundred pounds so far; her mom's down about fifty pounds. What have they done besides make changes in their eating habits? When I walk into the Lexington Athletic Club, I'm apt to see one or both of them sweating on a treadmill.

Have we helped changed Katie's future? As someone who spent much of her own childhood and adolescence struggling with weight problems, Diane hopes so.

Three weeks into the project, the church cook quit, and we suddenly inherited dinner for 120 people every Wednesday night, in addition to our dieters. We now cook for special dinners and Holy Week lunches and Vacation Bible School, and the Wednesday Night Dinners are averaging 175 people.

The recipes in this book are the result of feeding real people real food, night after night. They are the result of having real people say, "too spicy," "too dry," "too much," "too little." They were developed in the "test kitchen" at our church.

And while we were cooking, we were working on the book.

The Book

I started writing down my thoughts about our weight loss efforts when we'd been dieting for about nine months. I'd write a few pages on a subject, then put it down. A few days or a few weeks later, I'd write a little more. I've killed an incredible number of trees, and I'm not sure I ever thought my little scraps of ideas would actually grow up to be a *real* book.

We had a nice division of labor. Brett read all the technical stuff. I wrote prose. Diane was in charge of menu development and recipes. I fooled around, writing and rewriting, and eventually I actually produced enough words of prose to fill these pages. Diane kept creating recipes, and she finally had twenty-eight days of meals approved by our dieters.

Brett turned fifty in January 2004, and we wanted to have the book finished for his birthday. With the help of a local publisher, one friend who is an editor, and another friend who is a graphic artist, the first edition of the book was self-published, just in time for Brett's birthday.

Joseph Beth Booksellers, a local bookstore that has a policy of supporting Kentucky authors, agreed to carry the book and placed an order for ten copies. After an article appeared about us in the paper, that first order became three cartons. They scheduled a book signing, and suddenly our book was in a real live bookstore on its *very own* table. (Diane and I made several trips to the store to admire our book.)

While our book was on its very own table near the front of the store, Jennifer Crusie, a *New York Times* best-selling author, came to the store to do a book signing. She ended up with a copy of our book and really liked it. (That seems very reasonable. We have copies of all her novels in our basement, and we really like her books too.) She told her literary agent about our book, and that's how we ended up with an agent in New York City.

It's such fun to tell people the story of our book. What were the chances that we'd end up with an agent in New York? And that they would sell the book to Time Warner? So, I'm sitting here with another deadline. Making some changes, additions, and updates to the original book.

What happens next? I don't know; it hasn't happened yet. I'm talking about my own life here, and I want to flip to the back of the book to see where we end up. It's such an interesting feeling, and I have it a lot. Of course, by the time you're reading this, both of us will know what happens next. (I sure hope I like the last chapter.)

While we're waiting to see how the book part of the story ends, we're keeping busy. We've partnered with a local hospital to develop a weight management program that includes prepared food.

The Eucalorics Healthy Lifestyle Program

Cooking for our dieters at the church convinced us that Eucalorics, our theory of normal-calorie weight loss, had not only worked for us, but also worked for other people. What did we do now? What was the next step in our journey?

It was our dream to have the theories of Eucalorics become part of a weight management program that included health care professionals who could provide counseling in areas that Diane and I were not qualified to address. A partnership with Central Baptist Hospital in Lexington, Kentucky, is helping to make that dream a reality.

In the fall of 2004, a twelve-week, medically approved pilot program was conducted. Based on the favorable results of the pilot, the Eucalorics Healthy Lifestyle Program became a reality in January 2005. The hospital program includes counseling on diet and exercise from a nurse, a registered dietician, and an exercise physiologist. People's diet and exercise habits are reviewed. They have a fitness test and blood work. And professionals talk to them, not about dieting, but about making lifestyle changes. Permanent changes in their daily fare and their activity level that will allow them to become healthier, to lose weight, and to keep the weight off.

The recipes in this book, originally developed for the Temple Reconstruction Project, are being cooked every day, because the program includes the option of getting food. A registered dietician checked the recipes for the food we prepare before approving them for the program. (She also checked the book's menus and recipes.) People pick up a freshly prepared breakfast, lunch, and dinner five days a week. On the weekends, they have an opportunity to "practice" making changes for themselves.

In addition to their meals, we have a wide assortment of single-serving snacks, and everyone picks out their own discretionary calories. Then, out the door they go, with everything for the next day's meals all weighed and measured and packed in a little bag with the Eucalorics logo on the side.

When people are extremely overweight, their diets are tremendously out of control. Receiving their entire day's meals, based on the caloric intake recommended by the registered dietician, allows them to learn what nutritious, well-balanced meals look like. And what size portions will support a normal weight. Receiving meals means they get to see that it's possible to eat well and lose weight, and that successful weight loss does not have to mean eating horrible food and being hungry all the time.

Diane and I continue to cook. We design and develop recipes and plan menus. We look at "favorite" recipes and make recommendations to lower the calorie and fat content. We do a cooking demonstration once a month.

And most of all, we tell people there is hope. Even if you are tremendously overweight, there is hope.

CHAPTER 14

Changing Expectations

L et's compute the daily caloric intake that sustains your goal weight. Remember that we're using a rather low calorie factor based on an inactive lifestyle and a depressed basal metabolic rate. As you begin losing weight and increasing your activity level, you may need to add some calories to your diet. This will only become a great concern, however, if you start spending some serious time at the gym. It is estimated that a 150-pound person will expend 150–180 calories by walking *briskly* (3½ miles per hour) for 30 minutes. (This might be a good time to remind yourself that burning extra calories is only a small part of the benefits of exercise.)

Goal weight in pounds = _____

FEMALE:

_____ x 12 calories/pound = _____ calories
weight in pounds

MALE:

_____ x 14 calories/pound = _____ calories
weight in pounds

Take a look at the goal weight you picked. You probably picked that weight by asking, *What do I want to weigh?* Take a look at the number of calories that will maintain that weight, and ask a different question.

Is this a weight I can live with once I get there?

A weight *you can live with* means being willing and happy to eat the number of calories it takes to sustain that weight every day.

When I started, I picked 135 pounds as my goal weight, my *dream* weight. I use 135 pounds in all the calculations in the book. I use the calories it takes to maintain 135 pounds, about 1600 calories, as the number of calories I *try* to eat every day.

If you look at the menus and meals in this book, you see that my 1600 daily calorie intake allows me to eat very reasonable, nutritious meals. I'm generally happy with my food intake, but where does my 1600-calorie diet fail me? Discretionary calories.

Since my primary goal is to be healthy, most of my daily caloric intake is needed to meet the recommended consumption of fruits, vegetables, milk, meat, grains, and oils that my body needs to function well. There are very few calories left after I consume the foods recommended for optimal health.

Although higher daily caloric intakes do include more discretionary calories, they may not provide as many as you might think. If, for instance, you happen to have a daily caloric intake of 2000 calories, you're not supposed to be eating those "extra" 400 calories in junk food. Take another look at chapter 7. I'm supposed to be eating 6 servings of grains; you're supposed to be eating 7–8. I'm supposed to be eating 3–4 servings of vegetables; you're supposed to be eating 4–5. The recommendations for the nutritious food categories are all slightly higher for the 2000-calorie diet. And higher still for a 2400-calorie diet.

If you're overweight, you've been eating *some* extra discretionary calories. If, however, you're obese or morbidly obese, you've been consuming *lots* of extra discretionary calories.

What are we eating with those discretionary calories?

- A piece (or two) of birthday cake
- A pint of ice cream after a fender-bender
- A box of Valentine chocolates
- A glass of wine (or two) after a really bad day at work
- An anniversary dinner

- A few Christmas cookies
- A bag of M&M's when your husband breaks his ankle

If life didn't consist of special occasions and stressful events, it would be easy to get along without discretionary calories. But life is full of ups and downs, and my previous response to both the good and the bad things in my life was **FOOD**. What's my response now? Food.

I haven't changed my response completely; what I've done is alter the *magnitude* of my response. Will I ever think a birthday shouldn't include cake? I hope not. Will I ever become someone who responds to stress by losing weight? I doubt it. But my present relationship with food is healthier than it's ever been, and it keeps getting better.

I'm also realistic about needing to have more *extra* calories in my life. How do I increase my discretionary calories without increasing my weight? I pick up "extra" calories four or five times a week at the Lexington Athletic Club.

This book isn't about achieving perfection; it's about making improvements. It's about finding a sensible balance between your caloric intake *and* your basic metabolic needs *and* your physical activity that produces a weight *you can live with*. You may discover that somewhere between your present weight and your goal weight is the weight that ultimately makes both your mind and your body happy.

The Last Twelve Pounds

My previous weight of 247 pounds correlated with a BMI of 45.1 and the clinical definition of morbid obesity; my goal weight of 135 pounds correlated with a BMI of 24.7 and the clinical definition of normal weight. The journey from morbid obesity to normal weight represented 112 pounds.

How long did it take you to lose that much weight?

Well, it took a year and eight months to lose the first hundred pounds.

What happened to the last twelve pounds?

Can I let you know later?

There was something magical-sounding about losing one hundred pounds. But once I'd lost it, it became very difficult to get motivated to lose any more.

The loss of a hundred pounds put me at a familiar weight. A weight I'd been numerous times in my life. I might have no idea which single instant I weighed 110 pounds, but there had been a lot of days when I had weighed 147. Was this a weight my *body* was comfortable with or a weight my *mind* was comfortable with? I'm obviously eating a few more calories than my designated 1600, because I've stabilized at a slightly higher weight than my original goal weight of 135 pounds. Now, instead of being morbidly obese, I am one of those annoying women who complain about needing to lose ten pounds.

Have I learned to eat properly? I've certainly learned to eat tremendously better than when I started.

Will I lose the next twelve pounds? I'll have to get back to you on that. The dream weight is 135 pounds. It represents a 45 percent decrease in body weight. I'm hanging in there at 100 pounds lost, a decrease of 40 percent. Should I feel bad? I don't think so. Especially since I'm healthy.

Consider the Alternatives

You're almost finished with the first portion of the book. Do the ideas sound intriguing? Are you ready to jump right in on Day One? Ready to start looking at meal plans and recipes? Or are you overwhelmed?

You purchased this book, so you're obviously not happy with your weight. How unhappy are you? What else could you try?

YOU COULD DECIDE YOU DON'T CARE ABOUT BEING OVERWEIGHT

The anti-diet movement presents an alternative response to the widespread failure of traditional weight loss. Concerned with the psychological frustrations associated with continued failure, these groups focus on changing public attitudes toward the overweight population.

It is certainly true that in a country that strives to eliminate all forms of intolerance, discrimination against fat people is alive and well. A now famous article in the February 1994 issue of *Esquire* indicated that women between the ages of eighteen and twenty-five would rather be run over by a truck than be extremely fat. Two-thirds would choose to be mean or stupid rather than be fat.[22] The National Association to Advance Fat Acceptance (NAAFA) is one organization that lobbies against such attitudes. In an ideal world, no one would suffer from any form of discrimination, but the ethical stance that requires protection for the legal and moral rights of overweight individuals does not address the health issues associated with being overweight.

We live in a society that expects a legal solution to exist for every problem, but it won't help me to pass a law that makes it illegal to discriminate based on my weight if I die of a heart attack when I'm fifty-five. It's not possible to pass a law that mandates protection from the *medical* consequences of obesity. The morbidly obese, who have the greatest need of protection from discrimination, are also the most likely to have serious health consequences as a result of their excess weight.

Deciding you don't care about being overweight is ignoring the health risks associated with excess weight.

YOU COULD FOCUS ON MAINTAINING YOUR PRESENT WEIGHT

If you are *healthy* and overweight, deciding to maintain rather than lose weight may be the right choice for you. A recent publication from the American Medical Association designed to help physicians assess and manage adult obesity in their patients clearly views weight maintenance or modest weight loss as the best-case scenario for the average overweight and/or obese adult. The publication includes the following quote: "For many overweight and obese adults, achieving and maintaining a healthy weight is a difficult and lifelong process. For most overweight and obese adults, achieving a 'healthy' weight is an unrealistic expectation and should not be set as a goal. Improved health through improved weight or healthier weight in association with improved physical activity should be the goal."[23]

When might maintenance be the right choice? If you have no health problems associated with overweight, *and* you're physically fit, *and* you're perfectly happy with the number on the scales and the size on your clothing tags, who am I to insist that you should lose weight?

Hopefully, some of the ideas in the book will make maintaining weight easier.

YOU COULD DECIDE TO HAVE SURGERY

If you're morbidly obese, bariatric surgery is one possible solution to your weight problems. It was not a solution either Diane or I ever considered, although both of us would have been considered "good" candidates for this type of surgery.

The statistics for bariatric surgery are certainly better than the statistics for most diet programs, but they're still pretty sobering. The long-term prognosis following surgery indicates that you're not giving up food forever for *the promise to be thin*; you're giving up food forever for *a chance to be less fat*.

What do you get to eat after weight loss surgery? Take a look at the postsurgical diet of a gastric bypass patient.

Days 1–3: Intravenous liquids
Days 3–10: Clear liquids
- Low-sodium broth
- Sugar-free flavored gelatin
- Lemonade
- Fruit juice, except orange, pineapple, or tomato
- Decaffeinated coffee or tea

Days 10–17: Full liquid
Everything on clear liquid diet, plus:
- Cooked cereals
- Strained soups
- Skim milk
- Plain yogurt
- Orange, pineapple, and tomato juice
- Sugar-free pudding

Days 17–25: Pureed food
Everything on the clear/full liquid diet, plus:
- Pureed fruits and vegetables

- Pureed cooked meats
- Poached or soft-cooked eggs

Once you graduate to the regular diet, you can look forward to days with the following recommended food consumption:

8:00 a.m.
    1 egg (70 calories)
    ½ bread serving (40 calories)
    1 teaspoon diet margarine (15 calories)

9:15 a.m.
    4 ounces juice, consumed over 40–60 minutes (60 calories)

11:00 a.m.
    1 ounce skim milk (10 calories)
    1 ounce cereal (110 calories)

12:15 p.m.
    4 ounces skim milk, consumed over 40–60 minutes (45 calories)

2:00 p.m.
    ½ starch serving (50 calories)
    2 ounces lean meat or protein (60 calories)
    1 teaspoon diet margarine (15 calories)

3:15 p.m.
    4 ounces vegetable juice (25 calories)

5:00 p.m.
    ½ bread serving (40 calories)
    1 ounce lean meat or protein (30 calories)
    1 ounce vegetable (10 calories)
    1 teaspoon diet margarine (15 calories)

6:15 p.m.
    4 ounces skim milk, consumed over 40–60 minutes (45 calories)

8:00 p.m.
    4 ounces fruit (80 calories)

9:30 p.m.
    ½ bread serving (40 calories)
    1 ounce skim milk (10 calories)

If you total the calories, you'll discover that the bariatric surgery patient is subsisting on 770 calories a day.

If you are extremely heavy and learn to eat correctly, you will lose weight by making significant and permanent changes in your eating habits. If you are extremely heavy and have bariatric surgery, you will lose weight by making significant and permanent changes in your eating habits.

Yesterday, I ate 1540 calories. What did my day look like?

08:00 a.m.	Breakfast	Raspberry yogurt (90 calories)
		Orange (80 calories)
10:30 a.m.	Snack	Crackers and cheese (160 calories)
01:00 p.m.	Lunch	Greek salad, roll (320 calories)
03:30 p.m.	Snack	Teddy Grahams (160 calories)
07:00 p.m.	Dinner	Creole tilapia (110 calories)
		Andouille pilaf (200 calories)
		Stewed tomatoes (80 calories)
10:00 p.m.	Snack	94% fat-free popcorn (250 calories)
01:00 a.m.	Snack	Strawberry yogurt (90 calories)

Take a look at the menus in part 2 of this book. Take another look at a day in the life of a bariatric surgery patient.

Why do I think we'll be able to beat the statistics of both diet programs and bariatric surgery? We haven't lost weight by *going on a diet* and making temporary changes in our lives. We haven't lost weight by existing on the starvation rations of a post–bariatric surgery patient. We've lost weight by making permanent lifestyle changes.

I have more days that I do eat correctly than days that I don't, and I spend time on treadmills and elliptical trainers. I can go to New York and eat fabulous food, because I'll walk miles worth of blocks every day. I can choose to have cheesecake for dinner at night by spending an hour on a cross-trainer in the morning. I haven't given up eating normally forever in order to be *less fat*.

CHAPTER 15

Getting Started

It's time to take that goal weight, and translate *daily caloric allot-ment* into food. How do you decide what to eat?

If you're the average overweight female with a goal weight of 135 pounds, getting started is really easy. The meal plans are designed to meet your daily caloric intake of 1600 calories.

Each dinner recipe provides caloric and nutritional information based on ⅙ of a recipe, which is considered a "single-sized" portion. Daily caloric intakes close to the 1600 calories represented by the base meal plans will generally be single serving size. In order to provide sufficient calories for the higher daily caloric intakes, you may need to divide a recipe into four portions (multiply the caloric and nutritional information by 1½) and get a "1½-sized" portion. If you divide a recipe into three portions (multiply the calorie and nutritional information by 2), you'll get a "double-sized" portion. The guide below will help you decide which size portions *you* should be eating.

If you need to eat more than 1600 calories, make the following additions to the 1600-calorie meal plans.

1700 calories: Add a piece of fruit.
Adjust snack calories so total calories equal 1700.

1800 calories: Add a piece of fruit.
Add an extra serving of grain, i.e., a roll with dinner.
Adjust snack calories so total calories equal 1800.

1900 calories: Add a piece of fruit.
Add an extra serving of grain, i.e., a roll with dinner.
Adjust snack calories so total calories equal 1900.

2000 calories: Add a piece of fruit.
Add an extra serving of grain, i.e., a roll with dinner.
Have a 1½-sized portion of dinner.
Adjust snack calories so total calories equal 2000.

2100 calories: Add a piece of fruit.
Add an extra serving of grain, i.e., a roll with dinner.
Have a 1½-sized portion of dinner.
Adjust snack calories so total calories equal 2100.

2200 calories: Add a piece of fruit.
Add an extra serving of grain, i.e., a roll with dinner.
Have a 1½-sized portion of dinner.
Have an extra main course serving at lunch *or* an additional serving at breakfast.
Adjust snack calories so total calories equal 2200.

2300 calories: Add a piece of fruit.
Add an extra serving of grain, i.e., a roll with dinner.
Have a 1½-sized portion of dinner.
Have an extra main course serving at lunch *or* an additional serving at breakfast.
Adjust snack calories so total calories equal 2300.

2400 calories: Add a piece of fruit.
Add an extra serving of grain, i.e., a roll with dinner.
Have a 1½-sized portion of dinner.

Have an extra main course serving at lunch *and* an additional serving at breakfast.
Adjust snack calories so total calories equal 2400.

2500 calories: Add a piece of fruit.
Add an extra serving of grain, i.e., a roll with dinner.
Have a 1½-sized portion of dinner.
Have an extra main course serving at lunch *and* an additional serving at breakfast.
Adjust snack calories so total calories equal 2500.

2600 calories: Add a piece of fruit.
Add an extra serving of grain, i.e., a roll with dinner.
Have an extra main course serving at lunch *and* an additional serving at breakfast.
Have a double-sized portion of dinner.
Adjust snack calories so total calories equal 2600.

2700 calories: Add a piece of fruit.
Add an extra serving of grain, i.e., a roll with dinner.
Have an extra main course serving at lunch *and* an additional serving at breakfast.
Have a double-sized portion at dinner.
Adjust snack calories so total calories equal 2700.

2800 calories: Add a piece of fruit.
Add an extra serving of grain, i.e., a roll with dinner.
Have an extra main course serving at lunch *and* an additional serving at breakfast.
Have a double-sized portion at dinner.
Adjust snack calories so total calories equal 2800.

Table 15.1: Daily calorie allotments by meal

Calories	Breakfast	Lunch	Dinner	Snacks
1200	120–240	300–360	360–420	180–360
1300	130–260	325–390	390–455	195–390
1400	140–280	350–420	420–490	210–420
1500	150–300	375–450	450–525	225–450
1600	160–320	400–480	480–560	240–480
1700	170–340	425–510	510–595	255–510
1800	180–360	450–540	540–630	270–540
1900	190–380	475–570	570–665	285–570
2000	200–400	500–600	600–700	300–600
2100	210–420	525–630	630–735	315–630
2200	220–440	550–660	660–770	330–660
2300	230–460	575–690	690–805	345–690
2400	240–480	600–720	720–840	360–720
2500	250–500	625–750	750–875	375–750
2600	260–520	650–780	780–910	390–780
2700	270–540	675–810	810–945	405–810
2800	280–560	700–840	840–980	420–840
2900	290–580	725–870	870–1015	435–870
3000	300–600	750–900	900–1050	450–900

For caloric intakes greater than 2800 calories, snack calories continue to increase.

If your daily caloric intake requires fewer than 1600 calories, reduce your snack calories to reach the desired caloric intake.

The program is designed to be flexible. If you wish to switch any breakfast or any lunch or any dinner with the corresponding meal from another day, simply adjust your snack calories to compensate for the difference in caloric content of the switched meals. If you really liked the Barbecue Ranch Grilled Chicken Salad with Ritz Chips (total calories = 445 calories) from Day One, but you're allergic to the shrimp in the Mango Ginger Curried Shrimp Salad with Wheat Thins (total calories = 400 calories), simply switch the two meals and adjust your Day Ten snack calories down by 45 calories.

When you begin designing your own menus, Table 15.1 breaks daily caloric allotments from 1200 to 3000 calories into a range of calories for each meal as follows:

Breakfast: 10–20% total calories
Lunch: 25–30% total calories
Dinner: 30–35% total calories
Snacks: 20–30% total calories

You may notice that the maximums total more than 100 percent. This allows you to adjust your caloric intake to suit your lifestyle. (You obviously should not be eating the maximum percentage of calories for every meal and snack.)

Breakfast

Breakfast has been assigned 10–20 percent of my daily caloric allotment. I have a range of 160–320 calories for breakfast.

There's a good chance that you just thought to yourself, *Great, I'll have lots of calories for later in the day, since I never eat breakfast.*

How do I know that? In my former life, breakfast was the easiest meal to skip. I'm not a morning person, so I was always in a hurry. Besides, if I skipped breakfast I could bank those calories for later, right?

Ninety percent of the overweight population routinely skips one to two meals a day, and breakfast is the meal most commonly skipped.[24] But skipping breakfast is associated with overweight, rather than normal weight. Statistics indicate that the people who eat breakfast generally weigh less than those of us who don't eat breakfast.[25]

Why is skipping a meal counterproductive? First, when we do begin eating later in the day we overeat, more than compensating for those *saved* calories. Second, we sabotage our natural metabolic response to eating. When we eat, the body utilizes energy to digest, absorb, and metabolize the nutrients contained in the food. Dietary-induced thermogenesis, increased metabolic rate as a result of eating, reaches a maximum approximately one hour after a meal. Skipping meals tends to decrease our metabolic rate.

The greatest decrease in metabolic rate occurs during sleep. Breakfast literally means to "break a fast," and eating following the period of fasting associated with sleep provides a critical stimulus to the metabolism. The traditional wisdom that "breakfast is the most important meal of the day" is, therefore, backed up by present-day scientific knowledge.

The proverbial excuse for not eating breakfast is lack of time. Make time. There are many quick-and-easy, take-and-go options, and we provide some in the meals and menus section of the book. If you're serious about learning to eat correctly, the first absolute is breakfast. If you've never eaten breakfast, it's okay for breakfast to be a small meal. But something for breakfast is mandatory. If you're used to starting your day with 2 ounces of a high-sugar kid's cereal, you may be pleasantly surprised to discover that our dietician will ask you to start making changes in your diet by eating 1 ounce instead. She doesn't believe in asking people to change everything about their diet all at once; it's too much to expect. The nutrition profile for your day will look better if you choose a low-sugar, high-fiber cereal, but we don't expect your diet to be perfect on day one.

I'm still not a big breakfast eater. I don't eat as many calories in the morning as I probably should, but I always eat something. My stomach was initially quite surprised to get something besides diet Dr Pepper for breakfast. Now it expects it. It gets at least a cup of low-fat yogurt (and diet Dr Pepper).

Diane's better at eating breakfast than I am, but she's also significantly more alert in the morning. And really quite disgustingly cheerful. Since I'm usually awake long after she's fast asleep, I'm not nearly as charming in the morning as she is.

Lunch

Lunch receives 25–30 percent of my daily calorie allotment, or 400–480 calories. Since most of us aren't home to eat lunch, it can be a challenge to stay within this calorie window. If you pack a lunch, you're assured control over calories, but there is plenty of nutritional information available for eating out. Most fast-food establishments have information posted in the restaurant or on their Web site, and we've included a Fast-Food Guide at the end of the book.

Diane and I cook dinner five nights a week, but we frequently eat out at lunch. It is possible to achieve and maintain a normal weight while eating out, but you have to become an educated consumer. You have to know how many calories are in the food you are eating. And you have to be able to eat out without feeling deprived, or you'll create a situation that encourages overeating or bingeing because you're feeling sorry for yourself.

Dinner

For most of us, dinner is the main meal of the day. It receives 30–35 percent of the daily caloric allotment, so I have 480–560 calories for dinner. Whether I eat out or prepare a meal at home, dinner needs to be a meal, not an entrée. Dinner should consist of a protein, a starch, and a vegetable.

If you look at our menus, you'll notice that we plan meals. Why? In order to be physically healthy, we need to eat a variety of foods that contain the micro- and macronutrients our bodies need. In order to be mentally healthy, we need to choose our foods wisely, so we'll be getting enough food to be mentally, as well as physically, satisfied.

Snacks/Adjustments

This category receives a significant amount and the greatest range of calories, 15–30 percent. I've got 240–480 calories for either snacking or making adjustments to my other meals. This range of calories recognizes that in the world of eating, one size does not fit all. We have different lifestyles, different needs. We need to be able to have some flexibility in our meal and snack selection. These calories provide that flexibility.

If life were easy, we would make consistent food choices, so our bodies could be trained to eat approximately the same amount of food at the same time every day. But life is not always easy, and it can be hard to be consistent. We recommend trying to keep at least the pattern of your day consistent.

Try to eat a core number of calories at each meal or snack. Beyond the core calories, adjust additional calories to suit your particular lifestyle and pattern of eating. You know what time of day, and in what situations, you have problems with food.

These numbers are guidelines. Since each meal and/or snack is based on a range of calories, there is a great deal of flexibility in your caloric intake. Make the numbers work for you.

Do you need more calories at breakfast? If the high end of the range doesn't provide enough calories, add calories from the snack/ adjustments category until you're happy with your breakfast choices. Do you frequently eat out at lunch? Maybe you need extra calories there. Would it make sense for your dinner calories and lunch calories to be switched? Do you need to have an evening snack? Plan your day accordingly.

Depending on your beverage choices, you may need to utilize snack calories for calorie-containing beverages. The calories in sugared soda and sweetened tea can make those snack calories vanish very quickly. If you drink beer or wine, you'll need to pay attention to their calorie content. Alcohol is an energy source that provides approximately seven calories of energy per gram of weight when converted into glucose and metabolized. Diane had one friend who was quite unhappy to discover that bourbon and diet Coke wasn't a calorie-free drink.

Take a look at your own life and use the snack and adjustment calories to make the daily calorie allotment work for you. If you know you're going out for a special dinner, make *minor* adjustments in your daily schedule in order to compensate.

I find it is easiest to be mentally and physically happy eating 1600 calories a day if I eat consistently and frequently. I don't eat nearly as much at each meal, so I eat more often. A normal day in my life is presently divided as follows.

Breakfast: 100–300 calories
Midmorning snack: 100–200 calories
Lunch: 400–450 calories

Midafternoon snack: 200–300 calories
Dinner: 450–550 calories
Evening snack: 100–300 calories

There's an ongoing balancing act between getting appropriate nutrition and staying within the calories allotted to maintain your desired weight. The fewer the calories it takes to sustain your desired weight, the more difficult the balancing act becomes.

Do I Have to Count Calories?

We do. We keep a food journal, and we count calories.

The less you want to weigh, the more attention you have to pay to your caloric intake. You simply don't have enough calories, particularly discretionary calories, not to pay attention. If you're within ten or twenty pounds of weighing what you want to weigh, you need to have a really good grasp of the number of calories you're consuming in order to get to that lower weight.

If you follow our menus and use our recipes, a great deal of the calorie counting has already been done for you. We've given you twenty-eight days of meals. Twenty-eight breakfasts. Twenty-eight lunches. Twenty-eight dinners. They all have calorie and nutritional information.

The remainder of the book contains menus and recipes—practical applications of the theories and concepts we've been discussing.

Before you get started, do one last reality check. Have you picked a weight you can live with when you get there? Look at the number of calories that will sustain your goal weight and make sure it's a reasonable number. You're going to be eating it today. And tomorrow. In order to achieve and maintain the weight you've selected, you need to be happy eating this number of calories *forever*.

Beating the Odds

If you look at the statistics, it's remarkable that any of us ever bothers trying to lose weight. But there *are* people who are beating the odds. If you plan to be one of us, you need to begin your journey by accepting that we all *work* at keeping the weight off. It's not that we've purchased the secret to quick, easy weight loss that you haven't yet found; we work at staying at a healthy weight.

Start with realistic expectations. Don't expect exchanging bad habits for good habits to be a quick and easy process, and don't demand perfection. Simply believe that change is possible, and do your best. One day at a time.

What do we want for you? For you to look back someday at where you *were*, and marvel at where you *are*.

Every marathon starts with a first step. The loss of ten pounds or a hundred pounds starts with losing a single pound. Good luck.

Part Two

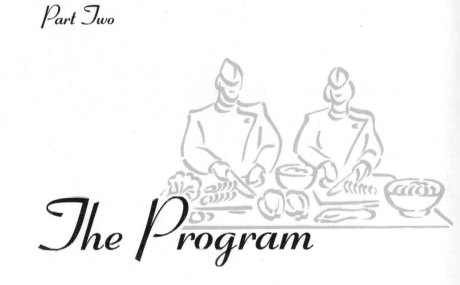

The Program

Day One

Breakfast

1 ounce bran flakes	(100 calories)
½ cup skim milk	(45 calories)
1 medium (5-ounce) banana	(90 calories)

Lunch

1 2-ounce French roll	(140 calories)
2 ounces lean deli honey ham	(60 calories)
1 ounce brie	(95 calories)
1 ounce baked potato chips	(115 calories)
1 small (4-ounce) Granny Smith apple	(70 calories)

Dinner

Honey Mustard Chicken	(230 calories)
Orzo Pilaf	(200 calories)
Roasted Asparagus	(25 calories)
1 cup skim milk	(90 calories)

Snacks

340 calories

Honey Mustard Chicken

6 PORTIONS

6	4-ounce boneless, skinless chicken breasts
	kosher salt
	black pepper
1 tablespoon	canola oil
1 tablespoon	unsalted butter
⅓ cup	honey
2 tablespoons	Dijon mustard
1 tablespoon	all-purpose flour
½ cup	fat-free, low-sodium chicken broth

Pat the chicken breast dry, then season with salt and pepper. Heat the oil and butter in a large skillet over medium-high heat. Brown the chicken in the oil and butter mixture, 4–5 minutes per side. Once browned, set the chicken aside.

In a medium bowl, whisk together the honey, Dijon mustard, flour, and broth. Add to the skillet and bring to a boil. Once the sauce thickens, return the chicken to the pan and cover it. Allow the chicken to simmer in the sauce over low heat until cooked though, 10–15 minutes.

Serving: 1 chicken breast with 1 ounce (2 tablespoons) sauce

230 calories
6 g fat
17 g carbohydrate
27 g protein

Orzo Pilaf

6 PORTIONS

1 tablespoon	unsalted butter
½ cup	orzo pasta (4 ounces)
1 cup	basmati rice (6 ounces)
1 teaspoon	kosher salt
½ teaspoon	black pepper
3 cups	fat-free, low-sodium chicken broth

Melt the butter in a medium saucepan. Add the orzo and basmati rice, and sauté over medium heat until golden brown, 5–7 minutes. Stir in the salt, pepper, and broth. Bring to a boil, cover, and cook over low heat until all the liquid is absorbed, 20–25 minutes.

Serving: ¾ cup

200 calories
3 g fat
38 g carbohydrate
5 g protein

Roasted Asparagus

6 PORTIONS

24 ounces	asparagus spears
	cooking spray
	kosher salt
	black pepper

Preheat the oven to 400°F. Wash the asparagus and trim the woody ends (the last 2–3 inches) from the spears and discard. Arrange the asparagus in a single layer on a foil-lined baking sheet. Coat the asparagus lightly with cooking spray. Roast 6–8 minutes, depending on the thickness of the spears. Remove from the oven and season with salt and pepper.

Serving: 3 ounces

25 calories
0 g fat
5 g carbohydrate
3 g protein

Helpful Tip
Thinner stalks of asparagus tend to be more tender and better for roasting.

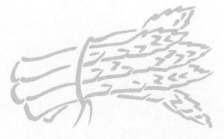

Day Two

Breakfast

1 3-ounce everything bagel	(235 calories)
2 tablespoons reduced-fat flavored cream cheese	(65 calories)
1 cup strawberries	(45 calories)

Lunch

Barbecue Ranch Grilled Chicken Salad	(315 calories)
1 ounce Ritz Chips	(130 calories)

Dinner

Meatloaf	(210 calories)
Buttermilk Mashed Potatoes	(130 calories)
Country Green Beans	(80 calories)
1 cup skim milk	(90 calories)

Snacks

300 calories

Barbecue Ranch Grilled Chicken Salad

1 PORTION

1	4-ounce boneless, skinless chicken breast
2 tablespoons	homemade or store-bought barbecue sauce
4 ounces	romaine or other dark leafy lettuce
¼ cup	scallions, sliced thin
1	Roma tomato, diced
1	large egg, hard-boiled and grated
3 tablespoons	Barbecue Ranch Dressing (see recipe that follows)

Coat the chicken breast with barbecue sauce, grill or broil until cooked through, 6–8 minutes per side. Slice the chicken into thin strips, then toss with the lettuce, scallions, tomato, and egg. Top with Barbecue Ranch Dressing.

315 calories
9.5 g fat
18 g carbohydrate
36 g protein

Barbecue Ranch Dressing

1 PORTION

2 tablespoons	*Ranch Dressing* (see page 148 for recipe)
1 tablespoon	*homemade or store-bought barbecue sauce*

Whisk together the dressing and barbecue sauce. Refrigerate at least 15 minutes before using.

35 calories
1.5 g fat
3 g carbohydrate
<1 g protein

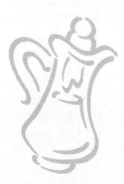

Meatloaf

½ cup	skim milk
1	large egg
½ cup	old-fashioned rolled oats (1½ ounces)
¼ cup	yellow onion, chopped (1½ ounces)
¼ cup	celery, diced (1 ounce)
1 teaspoon	kosher salt
½ teaspoon	black pepper
½ teaspoon	garlic powder
½ teaspoon	dry mustard
1 tablespoon	Worcestershire sauce
1½ pounds	96% extra-lean ground beef

Preheat the oven to 350°F. Stir together the milk and egg, then add the oats. Allow the mixture to stand for 5 minutes. Stir in the onion, celery, salt, pepper, garlic, mustard, and Worcestershire sauce. Combine with the ground beef, mixing well. Pack the meatloaf tightly into a large, 5-by-9-inch loaf pan. Bake uncovered for 50–55 minutes, until the meatloaf reaches an internal temperature of 165°F.

Serving: ⅙ of loaf

210 calories
6 g fat
11 g carbohydrate
32 g protein

Buttermilk Mashed Potatoes

6 PORTIONS

2 pounds	baking potatoes, peeled and chopped (6 cups)
1 tablespoon	unsalted butter
½ cup	1% buttermilk
1 teaspoon	kosher salt
¼ teaspoon	black pepper

Cover the potatoes with cold, salted water. Bring to a boil over high heat and cook until tender, 20–30 minutes. Drain well. Place in the bowl of a stand mixer. Add the butter, buttermilk, salt, and pepper. Whip the potatoes until smooth.

Serving: ¾ cup

130 calories
2 g fat
28 g carbohydrate
<1 g protein

Helpful Tip
If the potatoes will not be cooked immediately after peeling, cover with water and either the juice of one lemon or 2 tablespoons white vinegar to keep them from turning brown (oxidizing). Discard the acidulated water and rinse the potatoes before cooking.

Country Green Beans

6 PORTIONS

1 teaspoon	canola oil
1 cup	yellow onion, chopped (5½ ounces)
4 ounces	Canadian bacon, diced
24 ounces	frozen green beans
¼ teaspoon	crushed red pepper
1 cup	water
½ teaspoon	kosher salt
⅛ teaspoon	black pepper

Heat the oil in a large stockpot over medium-high heat. Sauté the onion and bacon until the onion begins to soften. Stir in the green beans, crushed red pepper, and water. Cover and allow the beans to stew over medium-low heat, stirring occasionally. After 1 hour, uncover the beans, and cook an additional 15–20 minutes until the excess liquid evaporates. Season with the salt and pepper before serving.

Serving: ⅔ cup

80 calories
2.5 g fat
10 g carbohydrate
6 g protein

> *Helpful Tip*
> "Seasoning": Canadian bacon is a great substitute for traditional cured bacon to cut back on fat when cooking southern-style vegetables.

Day Three

Breakfast

Fluffy Pancakes	(260 calories)
Blueberry Syrup	(120 calories)

Lunch

Egg Salad	(100 calories)
2 1-ounce slices white bread	(160 calories)
1 ounce fat-free pretzels	(110 calories)
1 large (4-ounce) kiwifruit	(55 calories)

Dinner

Linguine with White Clam Sauce	(310 calories)
Rainbow Carrot and Pepper Sauté	(50 calories)
1 cup skim milk	(90 calories)

Snacks

345 calories

Fluffy Pancakes

2 PORTIONS

1	*large egg*
⅓ cup	*skim milk*
1 tablespoon	*canola oil*
1 tablespoon	*granulated sugar*
½ cup	*all-purpose flour*
1½ teaspoons	*baking powder*
¼ teaspoon	*iodized salt*
	cooking spray

Combine the egg, milk, and oil. Sift together the dry ingredients, then stir in the liquid, whisking until smooth. Coat a large nonstick skillet with cooking spray, then heat over medium heat. Cook the pancakes in two batches, about 2 tablespoons of batter per pancake.

Serving: 4 pancakes

260 calories
10 g fat
34 g carbohydrate
8 g protein

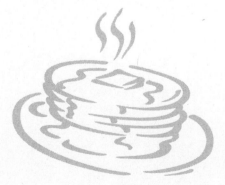

Blueberry Syrup

2 PORTIONS

¼ cup   water
¼ cup   granulated sugar
               pinch kosher salt
½ cup   fresh or frozen blueberries*
½ teaspoon   fresh-squeezed lemon juice

*Frozen mixed berries may be substituted for the blue-
berries.

Combine the water and sugar in a small saucepan with a pinch of salt. Dissolve the sugar over medium heat, then stir in the blueberries and lemon juice. Bring to a boil, then reduce heat to medium low. Cook 10–15 minutes, until the blueberries have popped and a bright blue syrup is achieved.
Serving: ¼ cup

120 calories
0 g fat
30 g carbohydrate
0 g protein

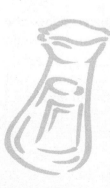

Egg Salad

9	*large eggs, hard-boiled*
3 tablespoons	*yellow onion, finely chopped (1 ounce)*
½ cup	*celery, chopped (2 ounces)*
½ cup	*reduced-fat mayonnaise*
1 tablespoon	*yellow mustard*
2 tablespoons	*dill pickle, minced*
1 teaspoon	*granulated sugar*
	kosher salt
	black pepper

Finely chop 3 whole hard-boiled eggs and 6 hard-boiled egg whites (discarding the extra yolks). Add the onion and celery. In a small bowl combine the mayonnaise, mustard, pickle, and sugar. Toss the dressing with the eggs. Season to taste with salt and pepper.

Serving: ⅓ cup

100 calories
5 g fat
4 g carbohydrate
7 g protein

Helpful Tip
Eggs that are 1–2 weeks old peel more easily after boiling than eggs that are fresh.

Linguine with White Clam Sauce

6 PORTIONS

2 tablespoons	olive oil
1 cup	yellow onion, chopped (5½ ounces)
3 cloves	garlic, minced
⅛ teaspoon	crushed red pepper
3 6½-ounce cans	chopped clams
3 tablespoons	all-purpose flour
1 8-ounce bottle	clam juice
12 ounces	linguine
2 tablespoons	unsalted butter
¼ cup	fresh parsley, chopped

Heat the oil in a large nonstick skillet over medium-high heat. Add the onion, garlic, and crushed red pepper. Sauté until the onion becomes translucent and the garlic begins to lightly brown.

Drain and reserve the juice from the canned clams. In a medium bowl, whisk together the flour and the reserved and bottled clam juice. Add to the skillet and allow the sauce to thicken. Stir in the clams. Bring a large pot of salted water to a boil. Cook the linguine according to the package instructions. Drain and toss with the butter before tossing with the clam sauce and parsley.

Serving: 1½ cups

310 calories
9 g fat
48 g carbohydrate
9 g protein

Rainbow Carrot and Pepper Sauté

6 PORTIONS

1 tablespoon	unsalted butter
1	large green bell pepper, cut into strips (5 ounces)
1	large red bell pepper, cut into strips (5 ounces)
1	large yellow bell pepper, cut into strips (5 ounces)
2 cups	baby carrots, shredded (10 ounces)
1 teaspoon	kosher salt
¼ teaspoon	black pepper

Melt the butter in a large nonstick skillet over medium-high heat. Add the pepper strips and carrots. Sauté for 5–7 minutes, until the peppers are tender and the shredded carrots are slightly limp. Toss with the salt and pepper.

Serving: ½ cup

50 calories
2.5 g fat
8 g carbohydrate
1 g protein

Day Four

Breakfast

1-ounce packet plain instant oatmeal	(100 calories)
1 tablespoon brown sugar, packed	(50 calories)
1 ounce dried cherries	(90 calories)
1 tablespoon toasted slivered almonds	(50 calories)

Lunch

Tuna Grinder	(310 calories)
1 ounce Doritos chips	(140 calories)
1 small (5-ounce) orange	(45 calories)

Dinner

Tamale Pie with Cornbread Crust	(400 calories)
Tossed Garden Salad	(35 calories)
2 tablespoons **Ranch Dressing**	(20 calories)
1 cup skim milk	(90 calories)

Snacks

270 calories

Tuna Grinder

1 PORTION

1 3-ounce can	solid *white albacore tuna,* *packed in water*
1 tablespoon	reduced-fat mayonnaise
	kosher salt
	black pepper
½	3-ounce plain bagel
½ ounce	cheddar cheese, sliced

Preheat the broiler. Drain the tuna well, then break up chunks into small flakes with a fork. Stir in the mayonnaise and season with salt and pepper. Spread the tuna mixture on top of the bagel half. Top with the sliced cheddar cheese. Place the tuna grinder on a baking sheet and place beneath the broiler. Broil for 5–7 minutes, until the cheese is melted and the bagel is browned around the edges.

310 calories
10 g fat
23 g carbohydrate
28 g protein

Tamale Pie with Cornbread Crust

6 PORTIONS

Chili Beef and Corn Filling

1½ pounds	96% extra-lean ground beef
1½ cups	yellow onion, chopped (8 ounces)
2 cloves	garlic, minced
1½ cups	frozen whole kernel corn (9 ounces)
1 28-ounce can	tomato sauce*
1 15-ounce can	petite diced tomatoes,* drained
1½ tablespoons	chili powder
1½ teaspoons	ground cumin
¾ teaspoon	kosher salt
¼ teaspoon	crushed red pepper (optional)

Cornbread Crust

½ cup	all-purpose flour (2.5 ounces)
½ cup	yellow cornmeal (2.5 ounces)
1 teaspoon	baking powder
½ teaspoon	iodized salt
½ teaspoon	chili powder
¼ teaspoon	ground cumin
1	large egg, separated
¾ cup	skim milk
2 tablespoons	unsalted butter, melted

*Low-salt and no-salt tomato products are now available. If you're concerned about sodium, these products are a better choice.

Preheat the oven to 400°F. In a large Dutch oven, brown the ground beef with the onion and garlic, stirring to break up the beef. When the meat is cooked, stir in the corn, tomato sauce, drained diced tomatoes, chili powder, cumin, salt, and optional crushed pepper. Allow to simmer 15–20 minutes.

While the chili beef and corn filling is simmering, prepare the cornbread crust. In a large bowl, whisk together the flour, cornmeal, baking powder, salt, chili powder, and cumin. In a small bowl, beat together the egg yolk and milk. By hand or with a mixer beat the egg white until soft peaks form. Stir the milk and egg yolk into the cornmeal mixture. Then fold in the egg white and finally the melted butter.

Place the chili beef and corn filling in the bottom of a 9-by-13-inch baking dish. Cover with the cornmeal batter. Bake for 25–30 minutes, until the crust is set and golden brown.

Serving: ⅙ of casserole

400 calories
10 g fat
49 g carbohydrate
37 g protein

Tossed Garden Salad

6 PORTIONS

12 ounces	romaine or other dark leafy lettuce
1 cup	baby carrots, shredded (5 ounces)
1	medium cucumber, peeled and chopped (7-ounce)
1	medium bell pepper, seeded and chopped (4-ounce)
1 cup	celery, diced (4 ounces)
1 cup	cherry tomatoes

Wash and dry the lettuce before chopping into bite-sized pieces. Toss with the remaining ingredients.

Serving: About 1½ cups salad

35 calories
0 g fat
7 g carbohydrate
2 g protein

Helpful Tip
The darker the green, the greater its vitamin and mineral content.

Ranch Dressing

12 PORTIONS

2 tablespoons	*ranch dressing mix*
½ cup	*reduced-fat mayonnaise*
¾ cup	*skim milk*

Whisk together the dressing mix, mayonnaise, and milk until smooth. Refrigerate for at least 20 minutes before using. The dressing will keep 2–3 days in the refrigerator.

Serving: 2 tablespoons

20 calories
1.5 g fat
<1 g carbohydrate
<1 g protein

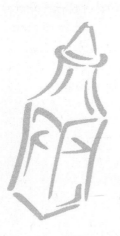

Day Five

Breakfast

Bacon and Cheddar Omelet   (250 calories)
Hash Brown Potatoes   (110 calories)

Lunch

Caribbean Curried Chicken Salad   (270 calories)
1 ounce Triscuit crackers   (130 calories)
½ cup pineapple chunks in juice   (70 calories)

Dinner

Barbecue-Rubbed Pork Loin   (180 calories)
Mustard Potato Salad   (150 calories)
Creamy Coleslaw   (70 calories)
1 cup skim milk   (90 calories)

Snacks

280 calories

Bacon and Cheddar Omelet

1 PORTION

	cooking spray
¾ cup	liquid egg substitute
	kosher salt
	black pepper
1 ounce	Canadian bacon, diced
½ ounce	cheddar cheese, shredded

Coat a nonstick omelet pan or small skillet with cooking spray and place over medium-high heat. Season the egg substitute with salt and pepper. When the pan is hot, pour the egg substitute into the pan and cook without stirring until the omelet begins to set and bubble up around the edges, about 15 seconds. With a spatula, lift the edge of the omelet to allow the liquid egg to run beneath it. Continue cooking until the bottom of the omelet is set, about 1 minute. Top the omelet with the bacon and cheese. Using the spatula, fold half of the omelet onto itself. Cook 1–2 minutes more, until the omelet is cooked through. Invert the omelet onto a plate.

250 calories
12 g fat
2 g carbohydrate
31 g protein

Hash Brown Potatoes

1 PORTION

1 teaspoon	*peanut oil*
½ cup	*fresh or frozen peeled and shredded potatoes*
⅛ teaspoon	*kosher salt*
	black pepper

Preheat oven to 300°F. Heat the oil in a nonstick skillet over high heat until almost smoking. Add the potatoes, salt, and black pepper. Cook, stirring frequently, until the potatoes are nicely browned, 4–5 minutes. Place in the oven to keep warm before serving.

110 calories
4.5 g fat
16 g carbohydrate
1 g protein

Helpful Tip
Peanut oil has a higher smoking point than either canola or olive oil so it produces a crispier product with less chance of burning.

Caribbean Curried Chicken Salad

6 PORTIONS

1½ pounds	boneless, skinless chicken breast
¾ cup	celery, diced (3 ounces)
¼ cup	green bell pepper, diced (1 ounce)
¼ cup	scallions, sliced thin
¼ cup	raisins
1 ounce	slivered almonds, toasted
1 clove	garlic, minced
⅓ cup	reduced-fat mayonnaise
½ cup	light sour cream
1½ teaspoons	curry powder
⅛ teaspoon	ground cinnamon
½ teaspoon	kosher salt
	pinch ground allspice
	pinch cayenne pepper (optional)

Place the chicken in a large saucepan and cover with cold water. Bring to a boil over high heat, reduce heat to low, and simmer for 15–20 minutes, until cooked through. Cool to room temperature, then cut or pull into bite-sized pieces.

Combine the chicken, celery, bell pepper, scallions, raisins, and almonds. In a small bowl, mix together the garlic, mayonnaise, sour cream, curry powder, cinnamon, salt, allspice, and optional cayenne pepper. Toss the chicken mixture with the curried dressing. The salad may be chilled for several hours or served immediately.

Serving: ⅔ cup

270 calories
9 g fat
9 g carbohydrate
38 g protein

Barbecue-Rubbed Pork Loin

6 PORTIONS

1	*2-pound center-cut pork loin*
1 tablespoon	*sweet paprika*
2 teaspoons	*granulated sugar*
1 teaspoon	*brown sugar, packed*
1 teaspoon	*onion powder*
½ teaspoon	*garlic powder*
1 teaspoon	*kosher salt*
½ teaspoon	*black pepper*

Preheat the oven to 325°F. Combine the dry ingredients. Pat the pork loin dry and rub with the barbecue spice mixture. Place the pork loin in the oven and roast for 50–55 minutes, until it reaches an internal temperature of 145°F. Remove it from the oven, cover with foil, and allow the meat to rest for at least 15 minutes before slicing and serving.

Serving: ⅙ of roast (approximately 4 ounces)

180 calories
4.5 g fat
3 g carbohydrate
31 g protein

Helpful Tip
The calorie/fat content of pork varies dramatically. Look for brands like Smithfield Lean Generation Pork, which contains 120 calories and 3.5 grams of fat per 4-ounce serving.

Mustard Potato Salad

6 PORTIONS

1½ pounds	red potatoes, unpeeled
½ cup	reduced-fat mayonnaise
1 tablespoon	yellow mustard
¼ cup	onion, chopped (1½ ounces)
¼ cup	celery, diced (1 ounce)
2 tablespoons	dill pickle, minced
2	large eggs, hard-boiled and grated
½ teaspoon	granulated sugar
½ teaspoon	kosher salt
⅛ teaspoon	black pepper

Cover the potatoes with cold, salted water. Bring to a boil and cook until just tender, 20–25 minutes. Drain well. Chill while preparing the dressing. In a bowl combine the mayonnaise, mustard, onion, celery, pickle, eggs, sugar, salt, and pepper. When the potatoes are cool enough to handle, dice into bite-sized chunks. Toss with the dressing. Serve immediately or chill and serve cold.

Serving: ⅔ cup

150 calories
4.5 g fat
22 g carbohydrate
2 g protein

Creamy Coleslaw

6 PORTIONS

24 ounces	coleslaw mix
½ cup	reduced-fat mayonnaise
2½ tablespoons	white wine vinegar
1½ teaspoons	granulated sugar
¼ teaspoon	celery seed
¼ teaspoon	prepared horseradish
½ teaspoon	kosher salt
⅛ teaspoon	black pepper

Combine the mayonnaise, vinegar, sugar, celery seed, horseradish, salt, and black pepper. Toss with the shredded coleslaw mix. (It will not look like enough dressing.) Cover and refrigerate for at least 30 minutes before serving.

Serving: ⅔ cup

70 calories
3 g fat
8 g carbohydrate
1 g protein

Day Six

Breakfast

Chocolate Chocolate Chip Muffins	(240 calories)
1 cup skim milk	(90 calories)

Lunch

Roasted Red Bell Pepper Hummus	(130 calories)
1 2-ounce pita bread	(160 calories)
Greek Tomato and Cucumber Salad	(100 calories)

Dinner

Chicken Cacciatore with Buttered Macaroni	(410 calories)
Tossed Garden Salad (see page 147)	(35 calories)
2 tablespoons **Creamy Italian Dressing**	(30 calories)
1 cup skim milk	(90 calories)

Snacks

315 calories

Chocolate Chocolate Chip Muffins

6 PORTIONS

2 tablespoons	Nutella Chocolate Hazelnut Spread
½ cup	granulated sugar
½ cup	liquid egg substitute
⅔ cup	all-purpose flour
⅓ cup	unsweetened cocoa powder
½ teaspoon	baking soda
⅛ teaspoon	iodized salt
½ cup	1% buttermilk
¼ cup	semi-sweet chocolate chips

Preheat the oven to 350°F. Cream together the Nutella and sugar. Stir in the egg substitute and beat until smooth.

Stir together the flour, cocoa, baking soda, and salt. Alternate adding the cocoa mixture and buttermilk, beginning and ending with the cocoa. Fold in the chocolate chips. Line a 12-cup muffin pan with paper liners. Divide the batter between the muffin cups, about 3 tablespoons per muffin. Bake for 22–25 minutes, until a tester comes out of the center clean and the top of the muffin springs back if pressed.

Serving: 2 muffins

240 calories
6 g fat
41 g carbohydrate
6 g protein

> *Helpful Tip*
> *Out of buttermilk? Substitute ½ cup skim or 1% milk mixed with 1½ teaspoons white vinegar.*

Roasted Red Bell Pepper Hummus

3 PORTIONS

1 16-ounce can	chickpeas, rinsed and drained
½ cup	canned roasted red bell peppers
1 tablespoon	fresh-squeezed lemon juice
2 tablespoons	olive oil
2 cloves	garlic, minced
1 teaspoon	kosher salt
¼ teaspoon	black pepper
2 tablespoons	fresh parsley

Combine all the ingredients in the bowl of a food processor. Process until smooth, adding 2–3 tablespoons of water if necessary. Refrigerate. Chill for at least 15 minutes before serving. Serve on pita bread.

Serving: ⅔ cup

130 calories
5 g fat
18 g carbohydrate
4 g protein

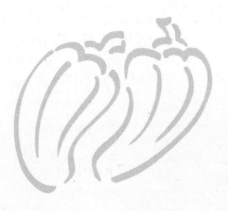

Greek Tomato and Cucumber Salad

6 PORTIONS

2 tablespoons	olive oil
1 tablespoon	red wine vinegar
¼ teaspoon	dried oregano
1 clove	garlic, minced
⅛ teaspoon	kosher salt
⅛ teaspoon	dried parsley
	pinch black pepper
1	large cucumber, peeled and chunked (10-ounce)
4	Roma tomatoes, quartered and seeded
½ cup	green bell pepper, sliced (1½ ounces)
½ cup	yellow onion, sliced (2 ounces)
6	medium black olives, pitted and sliced
2 ounces	feta cheese, crumbled

In a large bowl, whisk together the oil and vinegar, then stir in the oregano, garlic, salt, parsley, and black pepper. Add the vegetables and feta and toss until everything is well coated. Refrigerate for at least 15 minutes before serving.

Serving: ½ cup

100 calories
7 g fat
7 g carbohydrate
2 g protein

Chicken Cacciatore with Buttered Macaroni

6 PORTIONS

2 tablespoons	olive oil
6	4-ounce boneless, skinless chicken breasts
	kosher salt
	black pepper
1½ cups	yellow onion, sliced thin (6 ounces)
1	large bell pepper, sliced thin (6-ounce)
4 ounces	button mushrooms, sliced
3 cloves	garlic, minced
1 14.5-ounce can	diced tomatoes in sauce
1 15-ounce can	crushed tomatoes
1 6-ounce can	tomato paste
1½ tablespoons	dried basil
½ teaspoon	dried oregano
½ teaspoon	kosher salt
¼ teaspoon	crushed red pepper
8 ounces	macaroni
½ tablespoon	unsalted butter

Heat the oil over medium-high heat in a large Dutch oven. Pat the chicken breasts dry, then season with salt and black pepper. Brown the chicken in oil, 4–5 minutes per side. Place on a plate.

Add the onion, bell pepper, mushrooms, and garlic to the pan. Sauté for 5 minutes until the onion and bell pepper begin to soften and the mushrooms release their liquid. Stir in the tomato products, basil, oregano, salt, and crushed red pepper. Return the chicken to the pan and allow to simmer 25–30 minutes.

While the cacciatore is simmering, bring a large pot of salted water to a boil. Cook the macaroni according to the package directions. Drain well and toss with the butter.

Serving: 1 chicken breast, ½ cup sauce, ⅔ cup macaroni

410 calories
8 g fat
51 g carbohydrate
36 g protein

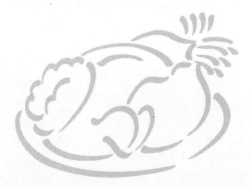

Creamy Italian Dressing

12 PORTIONS

⅓ cup	reduced-fat mayonnaise
½ cup	light sour cream
½ cup	skim milk
1 tablespoon	white wine vinegar
¾ teaspoon	lemon pepper
¼ teaspoon	garlic powder
¼ teaspoon	kosher salt
⅛ teaspoon	dried parsley
⅛ teaspoon	dried basil
⅛ teaspoon	black pepper
1 teaspoon	granulated sugar
	pinch dried oregano

Whisk together all the ingredients in a bowl. Refrigerate at least 15 minutes before serving. The dressing will keep up to 1 week in the refrigerator.

Serving: 2 tablespoons

30 calories
2 g fat
2 g carbohydrate
<1 g protein

Day Seven

Breakfast

6 ounces fat-free vanilla yogurt	(90 calories)
1 ounce granola cereal	(105 calories)
½ cup fresh or frozen raspberries	(30 calories)

Lunch

Beef and Bean Chili	(260 calories)
½ ounce shredded cheddar cheese	(55 calories)
8 saltine crackers	(100 calories)
1 cup mandarin orange segments in juice	(90 calories)

Dinner

Spice-Crusted Salmon Fillets	(220 calories)
Roasted Fingerling Potatoes and Fennel	(180 calories)
Sautéed Spinach with Onion	(35 calories)
1 cup skim milk	(90 calories)

Snacks

345 calories

Beef and Bean Chili

6 PORTIONS

1 pound	96% extra-lean ground beef
1 cup	yellow onion, chopped (5½ ounces)
2 15-ounce cans	kidney beans, rinsed and drained
3 tablespoons	chili powder
1 teaspoon	kosher salt
¾ teaspoon	ground cumin
¼ teaspoon	garlic powder
¼ teaspoon	dried oregano
¼ teaspoon	crushed red pepper
¼ teaspoon	black pepper
⅛ teaspoon	cayenne pepper, optional
1 29-ounce can	tomato sauce
1 14½-ounce can	petite diced tomatoes
2 cups	low-fat, low-sodium beef broth

In a large Dutch oven, brown the ground beef with the onion, stirring frequently to break up the beef. When the beef is cooked through, add the beans, chili powder, salt, cumin, garlic powder, oregano, crushed red pepper, black pepper, and optional cayenne pepper. Cook for 5 minutes, then stir in the tomato sauce, diced tomatoes, and beef broth. Allow to simmer 30–40 minutes before serving.

Serving: 1½ cups

260 calories
4 g fat
35 g carbohydrate
29 g protein

Spice-Crusted Salmon Fillets

6 PORTIONS

6	4-ounce salmon fillets, skinned with bones removed
2 tablespoons	whole cumin seed
1 tablespoon	ground coriander
1 tablespoon	whole fennel seed
1 teaspoon	kosher salt
½ teaspoon	black pepper

Preheat the oven to 350°F. Line a large baking sheet with foil. Place the salmon fillets skin side down. In a small bowl combine the cumin, coriander, fennel, salt, and black pepper. Sprinkle 2 rounded teaspoons of the spice mixture on each of the salmon fillets. Place the fish in the oven and bake for 20–25 minutes, until the fish begins to flake.

Serving: 1 salmon fillet

220 calories
10 g fat
1 g carbohydrate
29 g protein

Helpful Tip
Not familiar with fennel? It has a strong licorice flavor. If you're not crazy about licorice, leave it out of the spice rub and substitute 8 ounces of cauliflower for the fresh fennel in the next recipe.

Roasted Fingerling Potatoes with Fennel

6 PORTIONS

2 pounds	fingerling potatoes*
2 tablespoons	canola oil
1 teaspoon	kosher salt
½ teaspoon	black pepper
1 bulb	fresh fennel, sliced thin (8 ounces)
2 cups	red onion, sliced thin (8 ounces)
4 cloves	garlic, peeled and smashed

*Small red potatoes may be substituted if fingerlings are unavailable.

Preheat the oven to 400°F. Halve the fingerling potatoes. Toss with half of the oil, salt, and pepper. Place in a 9-by-13-inch baking dish and roast for 30 minutes. Toss the fennel, onion and garlic with the remaining oil, salt, and pepper. Add to the potatoes and roast for an additional 30 minutes, stirring once after 15 minutes.

Serving: ¾ cup

180 calories
4.5 g fat
34 g carbohydrate
1 g protein

Sautéed Spinach with Onion

6 PORTIONS

24 ounces	fresh baby spinach*
1 teaspoon	canola oil
½ cup	yellow onion, chopped (3 ounces)
¼ teaspoon	crushed red pepper
½ teaspoon	kosher salt
¼ teaspoon	granulated sugar

*Chopped, frozen spinach may be substituted. Thaw and squeeze the spinach to remove excess water before adding it to the Dutch oven.

If you're using fresh spinach, wash and spin dry before chopping into 1-inch pieces. In a large Dutch oven, heat the oil over medium-high heat. Sauté the onion until it becomes translucent, then stir in the crushed red pepper, salt, and sugar. Cook for 1 minute. Turn the heat to medium low and add the spinach, stirring occasionally until completely wilted, 3–4 minutes.

Serving: ½ cup

35 calories
1 g fat
5 g carbohydrate
3 g protein

Day Eight

Breakfast

1 ounce bran flakes	(100 calories)
½ cup skim milk	(45 calories)
1 medium (5-ounce) banana	(90 calories)

Lunch

1 2-ounce sourdough roll	(120 calories)
2 ounces lean deli smoked turkey	(60 calories)
¾ ounce Cojack cheese	(80 calories)
1 tablespoon **Santa Fe Sandwich Spread**	(25 calories)
1 ounce baked potato chips	(115 calories)
1 cup green grapes (5½ ounces)	(110 calories)

Dinner

Garlic and Pepper Pork Loin	(170 calories)
Cranberry Wild Rice	(190 calories)
Glazed Carrots	(60 calories)
1 cup skim milk	(90 calories)

Snacks

345 calories

Santa Fe Sandwich Spread

1 PORTION

1 tablespoon	reduced-fat mayonnaise
1 teaspoon	chili powder
⅛ teaspoon	ground cumin
	pinch kosher salt
	pinch black pepper

Combine all the ingredients in a small bowl. Allow the spread to sit for at least 15 minutes before using.

25 calories
2 g fat
3 g carbohydrate
0 g protein

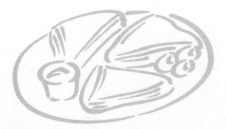

Garlic and Pepper Pork Loin

6 PORTIONS

2 cloves	garlic
1 teaspoon	black pepper
2 teaspoons	kosher salt
½ tablespoon	olive oil
1	2-pound center-cut pork loin

Preheat the oven to 325°F. Peel the garlic and use a mortar and pestle to mash the garlic, pepper, salt, and oil into a paste. Pat dry the pork loin and rub with the garlic and pepper paste. Allow the meat to marinate for at least 15 minutes and up to overnight. Place the pork loin in the oven and roast for 50–55 minutes, until it reaches an internal temperature of 145°F. Remove from the oven, cover with foil, and allow the meat to rest for at least 15 minutes before slicing and serving.

Serving: ⅙ of roast (approximately 4 ounces)

170 calories
5 g fat
<1 g carbohydrate
31 g protein

Helpful Tip
Trichinosis (the disease caused by a nematode found in pork) is neutralized once the meat reaches 137°F.

Cranberry Wild Rice

6 PORTIONS

1 tablespoon	unsalted butter
1 cup	yellow onion, chopped (5½ ounces)
1 clove	garlic, minced
¾ cup	basmati rice (4½ ounces)
⅓ cup	parboiled wild rice (2 ounces)
2½ cups	vegetable broth
1 teaspoon	kosher salt
⅛ teaspoon	black pepper
¼ cup	scallions, sliced thin
2 tablespoons	fresh parsley, minced
3 ounces	sweetened dried cranberries

Melt the butter in a medium saucepan. Add the onion and garlic, and sauté until the onion becomes translucent and the garlic begins to brown. Stir in the basmati and wild rice and cook 1 minute. Add the vegetable broth, salt, and pepper. Bring the broth to a boil, cover, and cook over low heat until all the liquid is absorbed, 25–30 minutes. Remove from the heat and stir in the scallions, parsley, and cranberries. Cover and allow the rice to stand 5 minutes before serving.

Serving: ¾ cup

190 calories
2 g fat
39 g carbohydrate
3 g protein

Glazed Carrots

6 PORTIONS

1 pound	baby carrots
1 tablespoon	unsalted butter
2 tablespoons	granulated sugar
½ teaspoon	kosher salt
	pinch black pepper

Bring a large pot of water to a boil. Boil the carrots for 10–12 minutes, until tender. Drain, reserving ¼ cup of the cooking liquid. In a nonstick skillet, melt the butter over medium-high heat. Stir together the sugar and cooking liquid. Add to the pan and bring to a boil. Add the carrots, salt, and pepper. Cook until most of the liquid evaporates and a glaze coats the carrots.

Serving: ½ cup

60 calories
2.5 g fat
10 g carbohydrate
<1 g protein

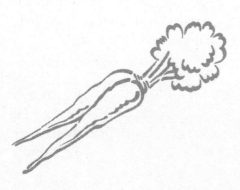

Day Nine

Breakfast

1 2-ounce cinnamon raisin English muffin	(150 calories)
½ tablespoon unsalted butter	(50 calories)
1 medium (5½-ounce) apple	(90 calories)

Lunch

Cobb Salad	(350 calories)
8 saltine crackers	(100 calories)
1 medium (5-ounce) nectarine	(65 calories)

Dinner

Ground Beef Stroganoff with Egg Noodles	(340 calories)
Green Beans with Carrots and Bell Peppers	(70 calories)
1 cup skim milk	(90 calories)

Snacks

295 calories

Cobb Salad

1 PORTION

1	4-ounce boneless, skinless chicken breast
1 ounce	Canadian bacon, diced
4 ounces	romaine or other dark leafy lettuce
1	Roma tomato, diced
1	large egg, hard-boiled and grated
3 tablespoons	Blue Cheese Dressing (see recipe that follows)

Grill or broil the chicken until cooked through, 6–8 minutes per side. Slice the chicken into thin strips, then toss with the bacon, lettuce, tomato, and egg. Top with Blue Cheese Dressing.

350 calories
15 g fat
9 g carbohydrate
44 g protein

Blue Cheese Dressing

6 PORTIONS

¼ cup	reduced-fat mayonnaise
¼ cup	light sour cream
⅓ cup	skim milk
1½ teaspoons	red wine vinegar
3 ounces	blue cheese, crumbled
½ teaspoon	dried parsley
⅛ teaspoon	garlic powder
2 dashes	Worcestershire sauce
	pinch kosher salt
	pinch black pepper

Combine the mayonnaise, sour cream, milk, vinegar, 2 ounces of the blue cheese, parsley, garlic, Worcestershire sauce, salt, and pepper in a blender or food processor. Process until smooth. Fold in the remaining ounce of blue cheese.

Serving: 3 tablespoons

90 calories
7 g fat
2 g carbohydrate
4 g protein

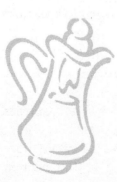

Ground Beef Stroganoff with Egg Noodles

6 PORTIONS

1 pound	96% extra-lean ground beef
1 cup	yellow onion, sliced thin (4 ounces)
8 ounces	button mushrooms, sliced
1 cup	2% milk
2 cups	low-fat, low-sodium beef broth
⅓ cup	all-purpose flour
1 teaspoon	Worcestershire sauce
1 teaspoon	kosher salt
½ teaspoon	black pepper
9 ounces	wide egg noodles
1 tablespoon	unsalted butter

In a large Dutch oven, brown the ground beef with the onion, stirring to break up the beef. When the meat is cooked, stir in the mushrooms and cook for 5 minutes, until the mushrooms begin to release their liquid. In a small bowl, whisk together the milk, broth, and flour, then stir in the Worcestershire sauce, salt, and pepper. Add the liquid to the pan and allow to come to a simmer and thicken, 15–20 minutes.

While the stroganoff simmers, bring a large pot of salted water to a boil. Cook the egg noodles according to the package directions. Drain well and toss with the butter.

Serving: ¾ cup egg noodles and ¾ cup stroganoff

340 calories
7 g fat
42 g carbohydrate
28 g protein

Green Beans with Carrots and Bell Peppers

6 PORTIONS

24 ounces	green beans, washed and trimmed
1 tablespoon	unsalted butter
1 cup	baby carrots, sliced thin (5 ounces)
1 cup	red bell pepper, sliced thin (5 ounces)
½ teaspoon	kosher salt
⅛ teaspoon	black pepper

Bring a large pot of water to a boil. Cook the green beans for 3–4 minutes, until tender. Drain well, then rinse immediately with cold water so the beans will not continue to cook. Melt the butter in a large nonstick skillet over medium-high heat. Add the carrots and peppers. Sauté for 5–7 minutes, until the peppers and carrots are tender. Add the beans to the pan and cook for 1–2 minutes to rewarm the beans and evenly distribute the carrots and peppers. Season with the salt and pepper.

Serving: ⅔ cup

70 calories
2 g fat
12 g carbohydrate
3 g protein

Day Ten

Breakfast

1 1-ounce packet instant cream of wheat	(100 calories)
½ tablespoon unsalted butter	(50 calories)
1 tablespoon brown sugar	(50 calories)
½ cup unsweetened applesauce	(50 calories)
1 cup skim milk	(90 calories)

Lunch

Mango Ginger Curried Shrimp Salad	(270 calories)
1 ounce Wheat Thins	(130 calories)

Dinner

Mushroom Smothered Chicken	(250 calories)
Smashed Parmesan and Roasted Garlic Potatoes	(170 calories)
Zucchini with Leeks	(40 calories)
1 cup skim milk	(90 calories)

Snacks

310 calories

Mango Ginger Curried Shrimp Salad

3 PORTIONS

1 pound	cooked salad shrimp
¾ cup	celery, diced (3 ounces)
¼ cup	green bell pepper, diced (1 ounce)
¼ cup	scallions, sliced thin
¼ cup	reduced-fat mayonnaise
¼ cup	light sour cream
3 tablespoons	Major Grey's chutney
1½ teaspoons	curry powder
½ teaspoon	kosher salt
	pinch cayenne pepper, optional

Combine the shrimp, celery, bell pepper, and scallions. In a small bowl combine the mayonnaise, sour cream, chutney, curry powder, salt, and optional cayenne pepper. Toss the shrimp with the curried dressing. Chill the salad several hours or serve immediately.

Serving: 1 cup

270 calories
7 g fat
14 g carbohydrate
33 g protein

Mushroom Smothered Chicken

6 PORTIONS

6	4-ounce boneless, skinless chicken breasts
1 tablespoon	canola oil
1 tablespoon	unsalted butter
½ cup	yellow onion, chopped (3 ounces)
1 clove	garlic, minced
½ cup	red wine
1 tablespoon	tomato paste
1 pound	button mushrooms, sliced
2 tablespoons	all-purpose flour
1 cup	fat-free, low-sodium chicken broth
1	bay leaf
¼ teaspoon	dried thyme
	kosher salt
	black pepper

Pat the chicken breasts dry, then season with salt and pepper. Heat the oil and butter in a large skillet over medium-high heat. Brown the chicken in the oil and butter mixture, 4–5 minutes per side. Once browned, set the chicken aside.

Add the onions and garlic to the skillet and cook, stirring frequently, until the garlic begins to brown and the onions become translucent. Deglaze the pan with wine and allow it to reduce until only a tablespoon remains. Stir in the tomato paste, then the mushrooms, stirring constantly until the mushrooms release their juices.

In a medium bowl, whisk together the flour, chicken broth,

and thyme. Add the mixture to the skillet along with the bay leaf and bring to a boil, stirring constantly until the sauce is thickened. Return the chicken to the skillet, turn the heat to low, and cover the pan. Allow the chicken to simmer in the sauce for 10–15 minutes, until the chicken is cooked through. Remove the bay leaf before serving.

Serving: 1 chicken breast with ½ cup mushroom sauce

250 calories
15 g fat
4 g carbohydrate
24 g protein

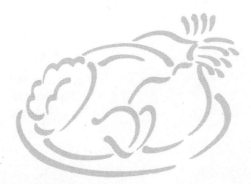

Smashed Parmesan and Roasted Garlic Potatoes

6 PORTIONS

1½ tablespoons	olive oil
6 cloves	garlic, whole
2 pounds	red potatoes, quartered
½ cup	fat-free, low-sodium chicken broth
2 ounces	Parmesan cheese, finely shredded
¾ teaspoon	kosher salt
¼ teaspoon	black pepper

Preheat oven to 375°F. Place the oil and garlic in a small ovenproof baking dish. Cover and place in the oven, roasting the garlic in the oil for 20–25 minutes until tender. Place the potatoes in a pot of cold, salted water and bring to a boil. Cook the potatoes until tender, 20–25 minutes. When cooked, drain well and return to pan. Add the chicken broth, roasted garlic and olive oil, Parmesan cheese, salt, and pepper. With a potato masher, smash the potatoes until the cheese is evenly distributed and potatoes reach the desired consistency.
Serving: ¾ cup

170 calories
5 g fat
28 g carbohydrate
4 g protein

Zucchini with Leeks

6 PORTIONS

24 ounces	zucchini
1	leek
1 tablespoon	unsalted butter
½ teaspoon	kosher salt
⅛ teaspoon	black pepper

Bring water to boil in a 2-quart saucepan. Depending on their size, either halve or quarter the zucchini lengthwise, then slice into 3-inch sections. Boil the zucchini for 3 minutes. Drain, and then rinse with cold water so they will not continue to cook.

Remove the stem end from the leek and cut in half lengthwise. Wash well to remove any grit from between the layers, and then slice the white part of the leek into half-moons. In a nonstick skillet, melt the butter over medium-high heat. Add the leek and sauté until it is tender, 3–4 minutes. Add the zucchini to the skillet and toss with the leeks. Season with salt and pepper.

Serving: ½ cup

40 calories
2 g fat
5 g carbohydrate
2 g protein

Day Eleven

Breakfast

1 cup low-fat cottage cheese	(160 calories)
½ cup canned peaches in juice	(55 calories)

Lunch

2 1-ounce slices pumpernickel bread	(150 calories)
2 ounces lean deli corned beef	(80 calories)
¾ ounce Swiss cheese	(80 calories)
2 tablespoons **Thousand Island Dressing**	(45 calories)
2 tablespoons sauerkraut	(5 calories)
1 ounce fat-free pretzels	(110 calories)
1 large (5-ounce) dill pickle	(25 calories)

Dinner

Black Pepper and Parmesan Shrimp Capellini	(380 calories)
Tossed Garden Salad (see page 147)	(35 calories)
2 tablespoons **Green Goddess Dressing**	(35 calories)
1 cup skim milk	(90 calories)

Snacks

350 calories

Thousand Island Dressing

12 PORTIONS

1 cup	reduced-fat mayonnaise
¼ cup	ketchup
2 tablespoons	sweet pickles, minced
2 tablespoons	sweet pickle juice
2 tablespoons	dehydrated onion flakes
½ teaspoon	kosher salt
¼ teaspoon	black pepper

Combine the mayonnaise, ketchup, sweet pickles and juice, onion flakes, salt, and pepper. Refrigerate for at least 15 minutes before using. Will keep in the refrigerator up to one month.

Serving: 2 tablespoons

45 calories
2.5 g fat
3 g carbohydrate
0 g protein

Black Pepper and Parmesan Shrimp Capellini

6 PORTIONS

1 tablespoon	unsalted butter
1 tablespoon	olive oil
3 cloves	garlic, minced
½ teaspoon	black pepper
1 teaspoon	anchovy paste
2 tablespoons	all-purpose flour
1 8-ounce bottle	clam juice
1 pound	cooked and peeled shrimp
12 ounces	capellini (angel hair) pasta
2 ounces	Parmesan cheese, finely shredded
2	Roma tomatoes, seeded and chopped
¼ cup	scallions, sliced thin

Place the butter, oil, garlic, and black pepper in a cold non-stick skillet. Over medium-high heat, melt the butter and cook the garlic until slightly golden. Stir in the anchovy paste and cook for 1 minute. In a small bowl, whisk the flour into the clam juice, then bring to a boil, stirring until it thickens.

While the sauce thickens, bring a large pot of salted water to a boil. Cook the pasta according to the package directions. Add the shrimp to the sauce to heat through. Drain the pasta well. Add the pasta, Parmesan cheese, tomatoes, and scallions to the sauce and toss to coat.

Serving: 1½ cups

380 calories
9 g fat
47 g carbohydrate
28 g protein

> *Helpful Tip*
> *Why a cold skillet? When the cold oil and butter are heated with the garlic and pepper, it infuses the oil and butter with their flavor.*

Green Goddess Dressing

12 PORTIONS

⅓ cup	reduced-fat mayonnaise
½ cup	light sour cream
½ cup	skim milk
2 tablespoons	fresh parsley
¼ cup	scallions, sliced thin
1 clove	garlic, minced
1 teaspoon	anchovy paste
1 tablespoon	white wine vinegar
¼ teaspoon	kosher salt
	pinch black pepper

Place all the ingredients in the bowl of a food processor. Process until the dressing is smooth and has acquired a pale green cast from the finely minced parsley and scallions. Refrigerate for at least 15 minutes before serving. The dressing will keep 2–3 days in the refrigerator.

Serving: 2 tablespoons

35 calories
2 g fat
2 g carbohydrate
<1 g protein

Day Twelve

Breakfast

2 1-ounce slices whole wheat bread, toasted	(150 calories)
1 tablespoon peanut butter	(95 calories)
1 tablespoon strawberry jam	(55 calories)

Lunch

Honey Pecan Chicken Salad	(300 calories)
1 1-ounce whole wheat roll	(75 calories)
1 cup red grapes (5½ ounces)	(115 calories)

Dinner

Pork Chops with Gravy	(190 calories)
Buttermilk Mashed Potatoes (see page 135)	(130 calories)
Country Green Beans (see page 136)	(80 calories)
1 cup skim milk	(90 calories)

Snacks

320 calories

Honey Pecan Chicken Salad

6 PORTIONS

1½ pounds	boneless, skinless chicken breast
2 tablespoons	honey, divided
1 ounce	pecan pieces
1 cup	celery, diced (4 ounces)
¼ cup	scallions, sliced thin
½ cup	reduced-fat mayonnaise
¼ cup	light sour cream
1 teaspoon	Dijon mustard
¾ teaspoon	kosher salt
	pinch black pepper

Place the chicken in a large saucepan and cover with cold water. Bring to a boil over high heat, turn heat to low, and simmer for 15–20 minutes, until cooked through. Cool to room temperature, then cut or pull into bite-sized pieces.

In a small saucepan, combine the pecan pieces and 1 tablespoon of honey. Cook over medium-high heat until the pecans are well coated and nicely toasted, about 5 minutes. Spray a pan with nonstick spray and place the nuts in a single layer. Allow them to cool, then break up any clumps that form. Mix the honeyed pecans with the chicken, celery, and scallions. In a small bowl combine the mayonnaise, sour cream, Dijon mustard, remaining tablespoon of honey, salt, and pepper. Toss the dressing with the chicken mixture. The salad may be chilled for several hours or served immediately.

Serving: ⅔ cup

300 calories
18 g fat
8 g carbohydrate
25 g protein

Pork Chops with Gravy

6 PORTIONS

1 tablespoon	unsalted butter
1 tablespoon	canola oil
6	4-ounce boneless, center-cut pork chops
3 tablespoons	all-purpose flour
½ cup	2% milk
	kosher salt
	black pepper

Melt the butter with canola oil in a large skillet over medium-high heat. Pat the pork chops dry and season with salt and pepper. When the butter and oil mixture is hot, add the pork chops, browning 5–6 minutes per side. Once browned, add 1 cup water to the pan and cover. Simmer the pork chops over medium-low heat until tender, 35–40 minutes. Once tender, remove the pork chops to a plate. Whisk the flour into the milk and add to the pork broth. Bring to a simmer and allow the gravy to thicken. Add salt and pepper to taste, then top the pork chops.

Serving: 1 pork chop with ¼ cup gravy

190 calories
8 g fat
4 g carbohydrate
24 g protein

Day Thirteen

Breakfast

Blueberry Muffins	(210 calories)
1 cup skim milk	(90 calories)

Lunch

1 2-ounce flour tortilla	(160 calories)
1 ounce lean deli honey ham	(30 calories)
1 ounce lean deli smoked turkey	(30 calories)
1 ounce lean deli roast beef	(30 calories)
1 slice 2% American cheese	(70 calories)
1 ounce baked potato chips	(115 calories)
1 cup strawberries	(45 calories)

Dinner

Chipotle Chicken	(155 calories)
Mexican Corn and Black Beans	(200 calories)
Tossed Garden Salad (see page 147)	(35 calories)
½ ounce Monterey Jack cheese	(55 calories)
2 tablespoons **Chipotle Ranch Dressing**	(45 calories)

Snacks

330 Calories

Blueberry Muffins

6 PORTIONS

2 tablespoons	unsalted butter, softened
½ cup	granulated sugar
½ cup	liquid egg substitute
1 cup	all-purpose flour
½ teaspoon	baking soda
⅛ teaspoon	iodized salt
½ cup	1% buttermilk
⅔ cup	fresh or frozen blueberries
1 teaspoon	lemon zest

Preheat the oven to 350°F. Cream together the butter and sugar. Stir in the egg substitute and beat until smooth. Stir together the flour, soda, and salt. Alternate adding the flour mixture and the buttermilk, beginning and ending with the flour. Fold in the blueberries and lemon zest. Line a 12-cup muffin pan with paper liners. Divide the batter between the cups, about 3 tablespoons per muffin. Bake for 22–25 minutes, until a tester comes out of the center clean and the top of the muffin springs back if pressed.

Serving: 2 muffins

210 calories
5 g fat
36 g carbohydrate
6 g protein

Chipotle Chicken

6 PORTIONS

⅓ cup	ketchup
2 tablespoons	light corn syrup
1 tablespoon	granulated sugar
1 teaspoon	brown sugar, packed
1 teaspoon	dehydrated onion flakes
½ teaspoon	dehydrated minced garlic
¼ teaspoon	ground cumin
⅛ teaspoon	chipotle chili powder
⅓ cup	tomato juice
6	4-ounce boneless, skinless chicken breasts

In a small saucepan, combine the ketchup, corn syrup, granulated sugar, brown sugar, onion, garlic, cumin, chipotle chili powder, and tomato juice. Allow the sauce to come to a boil over medium heat, stirring occasionally. Remove from the stove and allow to cool slightly. Remove and reserve ⅓ cup of chipotle sauce for the Chipotle Ranch Dressing (see recipe that follows). Use the remaining sauce to baste the chicken while broiling or grilling, 6–8 minutes per side.

Serving: 1 chicken breast

155 calories
1.5 g fat
9 g carbohydrate
27 g protein

Chipotle Ranch Dressing

6 PORTIONS

1 tablespoon	ranch dressing mix
⅓ cup	low-fat mayonnaise
½ cup	skim milk
⅓ cup	reserved chipotle sauce (from above recipe)

Whisk together the dressing mix, mayonnaise, milk, and chipotle sauce until smooth. Refrigerate for at least 20 minutes before using. Will keep 2–3 days in the refrigerator.
Serving: 3 tablespoons

45 calories
2 g fat
5 g carbohydrate
<1 g protein

Mexican Corn and Black Beans

6 PORTIONS

1 teaspoon	canola oil
1 cup	yellow onion, chopped (5½ ounces)
1 clove	garlic, minced
1 4-ounce can	mild green chilies
1 teaspoon	ground cumin
1 14½-ounce can	diced tomatoes, drained
3 cups	frozen whole kernel corn (18 ounces)
1 15-ounce can	black beans, rinsed and drained
1 teaspoon	kosher salt

Heat the oil in a large nonstick skillet over medium-high heat. Sauté the onion and garlic until the onion becomes translucent and the garlic begins to lightly brown. Stir in the remaining ingredients. Cover and turn down the heat to medium low and allow the mixture to cook 15–20 minutes. Uncover and cook 5–10 additional minutes, until the liquid evaporates.

Serving: ¾ cup

200 calories
2.5 g fat
38 g carbohydrate
10 g protein

Day Fourteen

Breakfast

Vegetable Frittata	(215 calories)
½ cup cantaloupe and ½ cup honeydew	(60 calories)
1 cup skim milk	(90 calories)

Lunch

Forest Mushroom Soup	(200 calories)
Swiss Toast	(180 calories)
Tossed Garden Salad (see page 147)	(35 calories)
2 tablespoons **Caesar Dressing** (see page 209)	(45 calories)

Dinner

Lemon Flounder	(140 calories)
Ham and Parmesan Orzo	(220 calories)
Garlic Broccoli	(45 calories)
1 cup skim milk	(90 calories)

Snacks

280 calories

Vegetable Frittata

1 PORTION

1 teaspoon	olive oil
2 tablespoons	yellow onion, finely chopped (½ ounce)
2 tablespoons	green bell pepper, finely chopped (½ ounce)
1	Roma tomato, seeded and diced
1 ounce	button mushrooms, sliced
¾ cup	liquid egg substitute
	pinch dried basil
	pinch garlic powder
	pinch kosher salt
	pinch black pepper
½ ounce	Parmesan cheese, finely grated

Preheat the oven to 350°F. Heat the oil in an omelet pan or small nonstick skillet over medium-high heat. Sauté the onion and bell pepper until the onion and pepper begin to color, 3–4 minutes. Stir in the tomato and mushrooms and cook an additional minute. In a bowl whisk together the egg substitute, basil, garlic, salt, and pepper. Pour over the vegetable mixture. Cook for 2–3 minutes until the egg begins to set. Sprinkle the top with Parmesan cheese and place in the oven. Bake for 8–10 minutes, until the frittata is cooked through and the cheese has melted.

215 calories
8.5 g fat
10 g carbohydrate
26 g protein

Forest Mushroom Soup

6 PORTIONS

2 14-ounce cans	low-fat, low-sodium beef broth
2 ounces	dehydrated exotic mushrooms (chanterelles, porcinis, shiitakes)
2 ounces	bacon, diced
1 cup	yellow onion, chopped (5½ ounces)
½ cup	baby carrots, chopped (2½ ounces)
½ cup	celery, chopped (2 ounces)
8 ounces	button mushrooms, sliced
2 tablespoons	tomato paste
½ cup	red wine
2 cups	2% milk
½ cup	all-purpose flour
¼ teaspoon	dried thyme
1	bay leaf
	kosher salt
	black pepper

Bring 1 can of beef broth to a boil in a small saucepan. Once it comes to a boil, remove from the heat and add the dehydrated mushrooms, allowing them to reconstitute for at least 30 minutes. Once the mushrooms have softened and cooled, place them in a food processor and puree.

Heat a large Dutch oven over medium-high heat. Add the diced bacon and allow the fat to begin to render. Once it has rendered and the bacon begins to color, add the onion, carrots, celery, and mushrooms. Sauté for 7–8 minutes, until the onion begins to brown. Stir in the tomato paste and cook for 1 minute before adding the wine. Bring the wine to a boil and reduce by half.

In a bowl whisk together the remaining can of broth, the milk, and the flour. Add to the pot along with the pureed mushrooms, thyme, and bay leaf. Bring the soup to a simmer and allow to thicken, 20–25 minutes. Season with salt and pepper to taste, and remove the bay leaf before serving.

Serving: 1½ cups

200 calories
8 g fat
26 g carbohydrate
8 g protein

Helpful Tip
Rendering refers to cooking meat products to release their fat. In this recipe, we render the bacon and use the resulting fat to sauté the vegetables, which allows the bacon flavor to pervade throughout the soup.

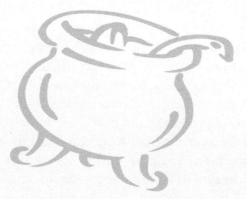

Swiss Toast

6 PORTIONS

1	12-ounce French baguette
3 ounces	Gruyère cheese, grated
	pinch ground nutmeg

Preheat the broiler. Split the baguette lengthwise. Divide the cheese between each half. Sprinkle lightly with nutmeg. Place under the broiler and toast until the cheese is completely melted and begins to brown around the edges.

Serving: 1/6 of baguette

180 calories
4.5 g fat
25 g carbohydrate
9 g fat

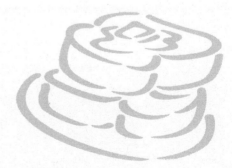

Lemon Flounder

6 PORTIONS

6	4-ounce flounder fillets
2 tablespoons	unsalted butter, melted
	kosher salt
	black pepper
2	lemons

Preheat the oven to 350°F. Place the flounder fillets on a baking sheet. Brush the fillets with butter and season with salt and pepper. Slice each lemon into 6 slices, and top each fish fillet with 2 slices. Place the fish in the oven and bake for 20–25 minutes, until the fish begins to flake.

Serving: 1 flounder fillet

140 calories
5 g fat
2 g carbohydrate
22 g protein

Helpful Tip
Cod, whitefish, or pollack can be substituted for the flounder.

Ham and Parmesan Orzo

6 PORTIONS

1 tablespoon	unsalted butter
1 clove	garlic, minced
2 ounces	lean deli honey ham, diced
1 cup	orzo pasta (8 ounces)
1 teaspoon	kosher salt
⅛ teaspoon	black pepper
⅛ teaspoon	lemon pepper
2 cups	water
2 ounces	Parmesan cheese, finely grated

Melt the butter in a large skillet over medium-high heat. Add the garlic and ham and sauté until the garlic begins to brown lightly. Add the orzo and stir until the pasta turns a golden brown. Stir in the salt, black pepper, and lemon pepper. Add the water and bring to a boil. Cover and turn the heat down to low. Cook for 25 minutes. Uncover the orzo and stir in the Parmesan cheese, cooking an additional 5 minutes, stirring frequently until the cheese is melted and the remaining liquid is absorbed.

Serving: ⅔ cup

220 calories
6 g fat
29 g carbohydrate
11 g protein

Garlic Broccoli

6 PORTIONS

24 ounces	broccoli florets
1½ teaspoons	olive oil
2 cloves	garlic, minced
¼ teaspoon	crushed red pepper
½ teaspoon	kosher salt
½ teaspoon	granulated sugar

Bring a large pot of water to a boil and cook the broccoli for 2 minutes. Drain, and then rinse with cold water so the broccoli will not continue to cook.

Place the oil, garlic, and crushed red pepper in a cold non-stick skillet. With the burner on medium-high heat, sauté the pepper and garlic until it begins to color and becomes fragrant. Add the broccoli, salt, and sugar to the pan and toss to rewarm the broccoli and coat with spicy garlic.

Serving: ½ cup

45 calories
1.5 g fat
7 g carbohydrate
3 g protein

Day Fifteen

Breakfast

1 ounce bran flakes	(100 calories)
½ cup skim milk	(45 calories)
1 medium (5-ounce) banana	(90 calories)

Lunch

2 1-ounce slices rye bread	(140 calories)
2 ounces lean deli pastrami	(80 calories)
¾ ounce Swiss cheese	(80 calories)
1 tablespoon spicy brown mustard	(5 calories)
1 ounce baked potato chips	(115 calories)
½ cup pears in juice	(60 calories)

Dinner

Chili Mac	(420 calories)
Tossed Garden Salad (see page 147)	(35 calories)
2 tablespoons **Thousand Island Dressing** (see page 185)	(45 calories)
1 cup skim milk	(90 calories)

Snacks

295 calories

Chili Mac

6 PORTIONS

1 pound	96% extra-lean ground beef
1 cup	yellow onion, chopped (5½ ounces)
1 cup	green bell pepper, chopped (4 ounces)
1 clove	garlic, minced
1½ tablespoons	chili powder
½ teaspoon	kosher salt
1 28-ounce can	crushed tomatoes
1 8-ounce can	tomato sauce
1 15-ounce can	diced tomatoes, drained
9 ounces	macaroni
4 ounces	cheddar cheese, finely shredded

Preheat the oven to 350°F. In a large Dutch oven, brown the ground beef with the onion, green pepper, and garlic, stirring frequently to break up the beef. When the beef is cooked through, add the chili powder, salt, crushed tomatoes, tomato sauce, and diced tomatoes. Allow to simmer 15–20 minutes.

While the chili mixture is simmering, bring a large pot of salted water to a boil over high heat. Cook the macaroni according to the package directions. Drain well. Toss the macaroni with the chili sauce. Place in a 9-by-13-inch ovenproof baking dish, and top with the cheddar cheese. Bake for 10–15 minutes, until the cheese is melted and the chili mac is bubbling around the edges.

Serving: ⅙ of casserole

420 calories
11 g fat
54 g carbohydrate
33 g protein

Day Sixteen

Breakfast

1 3-ounce blueberry bagel	(270 calories)
2 tablespoons reduced-fat strawberry cream cheese	(60 calories)

Lunch

Grilled Chicken Caesar Salad	(280 calories)
1 2-ounce sourdough roll	(120 calories)

Dinner

Ham and Egg Fried Rice	(320 calories)
Sesame Hoisin Green Beans	(100 calories)
1 cup skim milk	(90 calories)

Snacks

360 calories

Grilled Chicken Caesar Salad

1 PORTION

1	4-ounce boneless, skinless chicken breast
4 ounces	romaine lettuce
3 tablespoons	Caesar Dressing (see recipe that follows)
½ ounce	Parmesan cheese, finely shredded

Grill or broil the chicken until cooked through, 6–8 minutes per side. Toss the lettuce with dressing until well coated. Slice chicken into thin strips and top lettuce with it and the Parmesan cheese.

280 calories
10.5 g fat
5 g carbohydrate
38 g protein

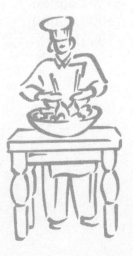

Caesar Dressing

8 PORTIONS

⅓ cup	reduced-fat mayonnaise
¼ cup	light sour cream
½ cup	skim milk
1 tablespoon	fresh-squeezed lemon juice
3 cloves	garlic, mashed to a paste
1 teaspoon	anchovy paste
¼ teaspoon	kosher salt
½ teaspoon	black pepper
2 ounces	Parmesan cheese, finely grated

Combine all ingredients. Refrigerate at least 15 minutes before using. Caesar dressing will keep 2–3 days in the refrigerator.
Serving: 3 tablespoons

70 calories
4.5 g fat
2 g carbohydrate
4 g protein

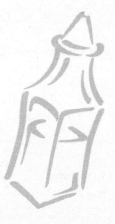

Ham and Egg Fried Rice

6 PORTIONS

3 tablespoons	canola oil
3	large eggs, beaten
6 ounces	lean ham, diced
¾ cup	yellow onion, chopped (4 ounces)
⅓ cup	frozen peas (1½ ounces)
⅓ cup	baby carrots, diced (1½ ounces)
4½ cups	basmati rice, cooked (24 ounces)
⅓ cup	low sodium soy sauce
⅜ teaspoon	white pepper

Heat 1 tablespoon of the oil in a large nonstick skillet over medium-high heat. Add the eggs and scramble until completely cooked. Set aside on a plate.

Heat the remaining 2 tablespoons of oil. Add the ham, onion, peas, and carrots and cook 1 minute. Stir in the rice, soy sauce, and white pepper. Stir the rice frequently, until the vegetables are tender and the rice is crisp, 5–7 minutes. Return the egg to the skillet and fold in until distributed throughout the fried rice.

Serving: 1 generous cup

320 calories
13 g fat
38 g carbohydrate
12 g protein

Helpful Tip
Basmati rice when cooked yields 3 cups for every cup raw. To yield 4½ cups cooked rice requires 1½ cups raw rice.

Sesame Hoisin Green Beans

6 PORTIONS

24 ounces	green beans, washed and trimmed
1 tablespoon	canola oil
1½ teaspoons	toasted sesame oil
3 tablespoons	hoisin sauce
1½ tablespoons	low-sodium soy sauce
1½ teaspoons	chili-garlic sauce
1½ teaspoons	granulated sugar
4 tablespoons	water
1½ tablespoons	cornstarch
½ cup	scallions, sliced thin

Bring a large pot of water to a boil. Boil the beans until tender crisp, 3–4 minutes. Drain well, and then rinse immediately with cold water so the beans will not continue to cook.

In a bowl combine all the remaining ingredients except the scallions. Warm a large skillet over medium-high heat. Add the sauce ingredients and bring them to a boil. When the sauce thickens, add the green beans, tossing to coat. Remove from the heat and garnish with the scallions.

Serving: ½ cup

100 calories
4 g fat
15 g carbohydrate
3 g protein

Day Seventeen

Breakfast

1-ounce packet plain instant oatmeal	(100 calories)
1 tablespoon brown sugar, packed	(50 calories)
1 ounce dried cranberries	(90 calories)
1 tablespoon toasted walnut pieces	(50 calories)

Lunch

Italian Ham and Provolone Melt	(360 calories)
½ cup honeydew and ½ cup cantaloupe	(60 calories)

Dinner

Spaghetti with Meat Sauce	(430 calories)
Tossed Garden Salad (see page 147)	(35 calories)
2 tablespoons **Creamy Italian Dressing** (see page 162)	(30 calories)
1 cup skim milk	(90 calories)

Snacks

305 calories

Italian Ham and Provolone Melt

1 PORTION

1	2-ounce Italian roll
½ tablespoon	unsalted butter
	pinch garlic powder
2 ounces	lean deli ham
¾ ounce	provolone cheese
1	Roma tomato, sliced
	pinch dried basil

Preheat the broiler. Spread the roll with butter and sprinkle with garlic powder. Top one-half with the ham, then the cheese and tomato. Sprinkle with basil. Place both halves beneath the broiler and toast until the cheese is melted and the bread begins to brown.

360 calories
16 g fat
32 g carbohydrate
22 g protein

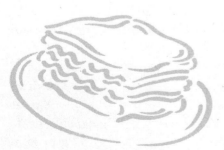

Spaghetti with Meat Sauce

6 PORTIONS

1 pound	96% extra-lean ground beef
½ cup	yellow onion, chopped (3 ounces)
3 cloves	garlic, minced
1 28-ounce can	crushed tomatoes
1 8-ounce can	tomato sauce
1 cup	low-fat, low-sodium beef broth
1 teaspoon	dried basil
½ teaspoon	dried oregano
¼ teaspoon	dried thyme
¼ teaspoon	kosher salt
⅛ teaspoon	crushed red pepper
12 ounces	thin spaghetti
3 ounces	Parmesan cheese, finely shredded

In a large Dutch oven, brown the ground beef, onion, and garlic over medium-high heat, stirring to break up the meat. When the meat is cooked, add the crushed tomatoes, tomato sauce, broth, basil, oregano, thyme, salt, and crushed red pepper. Allow to simmer at least 15 minutes.

Bring a large pot of salted water to a boil. Cook the spaghetti according to the package directions. Drain the pasta well before serving with the spaghetti sauce.

Serving: 1 cup pasta, 1 cup sauce, 2 tablespoons Parmesan cheese

430 calories
8 g fat
58 g carbohydrate
37 g protein

Day Eighteen

Breakfast

1 3-ounce plain bagel, toasted	(230 calories)
Cinnamon Sugar Spread	(100 calories)

Lunch

Corn and Crab Pasta Salad	(310 calories)
1 cup green grapes (5½ ounces)	(115 calories)

Dinner

Chicken and French Onion Risotto	(370 calories)
Roasted Asparagus (see page 130)	(25 calories)
1 cup skim milk	(90 calories)

Snacks

360 calories

Cinnamon Sugar Spread

1 PORTION

½ tablespoon   unsalted butter, softened
1 tablespoon   brown sugar, packed
⅛ teaspoon   ground cinnamon

Combine the butter, sugar, and cinnamon until a smooth spread is achieved. Use to top bagels, toast, or English muffins before toasting.

100 calories
6 g fat
14 g carbohydrate
0 g protein

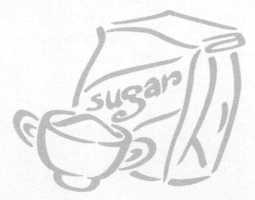

Corn and Crab Pasta Salad

6 PORTIONS

1½ cups	frozen whole kernel corn (9 ounces)
8 ounces	penne pasta
1 pound	cooked claw crabmeat
¾ cup	celery, diced (3 ounces)
¾ cup	red bell pepper, diced (3 ounces)
⅓ cup	scallions, sliced thin
1 cup	reduced-fat mayonnaise
1 cup	light sour cream
1 tablespoon	Old Bay seasoning
½ teaspoon	kosher salt
	pinch black pepper

Microwave the corn for 5 minutes, to thaw and cook slightly. Set aside and allow to cool. Bring a large pot of salted water to a boil over high heat. Cook the penne according to the package directions, then drain and rinse with cold water. Pick over the crab to check for any pieces of shell. Combine the crab with the corn, celery, red bell pepper, and scallions. In a small bowl combine the mayonnaise, sour cream, Old Bay seasoning, salt, and pepper. Combine with the crab mixture and penne. The salad may be chilled for several hours, or served immediately.

Serving: 1½ cups

310 calories
12 g fat
25 g carbohydrate
21 g protein

Chicken and French Onion Risotto

6 PORTIONS

1½ pounds	boneless, skinless chicken breast
3 cups	fat-free, low-sodium chicken broth
1 tablespoon	unsalted butter
2 tablespoons	olive oil
3 cups	yellow onion, sliced thin (12 ounces)
2 cloves	garlic, minced
1 teaspoon	granulated sugar
½ teaspoon	kosher salt
¼ teaspoon	black pepper
1 cup	arborio rice (6 ounces)
1 cup	white wine
1½ ounces	Parmesan cheese, finely shredded
1½ ounces	Gruyère cheese, finely shredded

Place the chicken in a large saucepan and cover with the cold chicken broth. Bring to a boil over high heat, then turn to low and simmer the chicken for 15–20 minutes, until cooked through. Cut into bite-sized pieces. With a fine wire mesh strainer, skim off any scum left behind in the chicken broth and reserve for the risotto.

While the chicken is poaching, melt the butter with the oil over medium heat in a large skillet. Add the onion, garlic, sugar, salt, and pepper. Cover and cook 5 minutes, allowing the onions to start sweating. Uncover and continue to cook the onions until they caramelize, 20–25 minutes more.

Once the onions are a deep golden brown, add the rice and cook for 1 minute before stirring in the wine. Stirring frequently, allow the wine to come to a boil and reduce almost completely. Once the wine is evaporated, add 1 cup of broth to the rice. Stir frequently and allow it to simmer and be completely absorbed. Once the first cup of broth is absorbed, add the second. Again stir frequently until the second cup is absorbed before adding the remaining broth. When nearly all of the final broth is absorbed, add the chicken and the Parmesan and Gruyère cheese, stirring until the cheese is melted and fully incorporated into the risotto.

Serving: 1½ cups

370 calories
13 g fat
29 g carbohydrate
34 g protein

Helpful Tip
What's the white stuff in the broth? Protein particles that co-agulated during the cooking process. They won't hurt the taste of the finished product but are unpleasant-looking and simple to strain out.

Day Nineteen

Breakfast

Huevos Rancheros   (280 calories)
1 cup pineapple chunks in juice   (140 calories)

Lunch

Traditional Chicken Salad   (190 calories)
1 2-ounce sourdough roll   (120 calories)
1 cup cherry tomatoes   (30 calories)

Dinner

Andouille and Crawfish Trinity   (160 calories)
Scallion and Parsley Pilaf   (190 calories)
Garlic Zucchini   (35 calories)
1 cup skim milk   (90 calories)

Snacks

365 calories

Huevos Rancheros

1 PORTION

	cooking spray
½ cup	*liquid egg substitute*
1	*1-ounce flour tortilla*
½ ounce	*Mexican-blend cheese, shredded*
2 tablespoons	*salsa*

Coat a small nonstick skillet with cooking spray and heat over medium-high heat. When the pan is hot, add the eggs and scramble until cooked through. Place the eggs in the center of the tortilla and top with cheese and salsa. Roll like a burrito.

280 calories
12 g fat
21 g carbohydrate
22 g protein

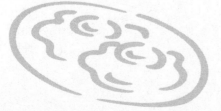

Traditional Chicken Salad

6 PORTIONS

1½ pounds	boneless, skinless chicken breast
⅔ cup	red grapes, halved
¾ cup	celery, diced (3 ounces)
¼ cup	scallions, sliced thin
½ cup	reduced-fat mayonnaise
¼ cup	light sour cream
¾ teaspoon	kosher salt
½ teaspoon	granulated sugar
¼ teaspoon	poultry seasoning
⅛ teaspoon	black pepper

Place the chicken in a large saucepan and cover with cold water. Bring to a boil over high heat, turn heat to low, and simmer for 15–20 minutes, until cooked through. Cool to room temperature, then cut or pull into bite-sized pieces.

Combine the chicken, grapes, celery, and scallions in a large bowl. In a separate bowl, stir together the mayonnaise, sour cream, salt, sugar, poultry seasoning, and black pepper. Toss the dressing with the chicken mixture. The salad may be chilled several hours or served immediately.

Serving: ⅔ cup

190 calories
5 g fat
5 g carbohydrate
27 g protein

Andouille and Crawfish Trinity

6 PORTIONS

4 ounces	andouille sausage
2 cloves	garlic, minced
½ cup	yellow onion, chopped (3 ounces)
½ cup	celery, chopped (2 ounces)
½ cup	green bell pepper, chopped (2 ounces)
2 teaspoons	dried basil
1 teaspoon	dried thyme
½ teaspoon	sweet paprika
2 8-ounce bottles	clam juice
3 tablespoons	all-purpose flour
1 pound	cooked crawfish tailmeat*

*Shrimp may be substituted for the crawfish.

Quarter the andouille sausage lengthwise, then cut into quarter-inch slices. Place in a large nonstick skillet and brown over medium-high heat. After the fat has begun to render, 2–3 minutes, add the garlic, onion, celery, and bell pepper. Cook until the vegetable trinity begins to soften and the garlic begins to brown. Stir in the basil, thyme, and paprika. Whisk together the clam juice and flour, then add to the pan and allow to come to a boil and thicken. When the sauce is thickened and smooth, stir in the crawfish to heat through. Serve over Scallion and Parsley Pilaf (see recipe that follows).

Serving: ¾ cup

160 calories
6 g fat

6 g carbohydrate
19 g protein

> *Helpful Tip*
> Andouille sausage is a spicy garlic smoked sausage used in Cajun cooking. It is becoming widely available, but any good smoked sausage will do.

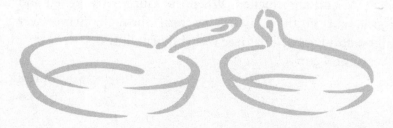

Scallion and Parsley Pilaf

6 PORTIONS

1 tablespoon	unsalted butter
1½ cups	basmati rice (9 ounces)
1 teaspoon	kosher salt
⅛ teaspoon	black pepper
3 cups	water
¼ cup	fresh parsley, minced
¼ cup	scallions, sliced thin

Melt the butter in a large skillet over medium-high heat. Add the rice to the pan and sauté until it browns slightly, 4–5 minutes. Stir in the salt, pepper, and water. Bring to a boil, cover, and turn the heat to low. When the liquid has been absorbed, 20–25 minutes, stir in the parsley and scallions.

Serving: ¾ cup

190 calories
3 g fat
35 g carbohydrate
6 g protein

> *Helpful Tip*
> *Parsley will stay fresh longer if stored in the refrigerator in a glass of water.*

Garlic Zucchini

6 PORTIONS

24 ounces	zucchini
1 tablespoon	unsalted butter
3 cloves	garlic, minced
½ teaspoon	kosher salt
⅛ teaspoon	black pepper

Bring water to a boil in a 2-quart saucepan. Depending on their size either halve or quarter the zucchini lengthwise, then slice into 3-inch sections. Boil for 3 minutes. Drain, and then rinse with cold water so the zucchini will not continue to cook.

In a nonstick skillet, melt the butter over medium-high heat. Add the garlic, salt, and pepper. Sauté the garlic until it is fragrant. Add the zucchini and toss to distribute the garlic butter.

Serving: ½ cup

35 calories
2 g fat
4 g carbohydrate
1 g protein

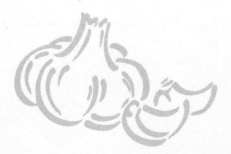

Day Twenty

Breakfast

Cinnamon Raisin Pull-Aparts	(210 calories)
1 cup skim milk	(90 calories)

Lunch

Soft Bean Burrito	(440 calories)
1 medium (7-ounce) orange	(90 calories)

Dinner

Barbecue Chicken	(180 calories)
Cheddar and Chive Mashed Potatoes	(170 calories)
Green Beans with Red Onion and Red Pepper	(60 calories)
1 cup skim milk	(90 calories)

Snacks

270 calories

Cinnamon Raisin Pull-Aparts

5 PORTIONS

	cooking spray
½ teaspoon	ground cinnamon
⅓ cup	brown sugar, packed
1 7½-ounce can	Pillsbury buttermilk biscuits
2 tablespoons	unsalted butter, melted
2 tablespoons	raisins

Preheat the oven to 350°F. Coat a 6-cup muffin pan with cooking spray. Combine the cinnamon and sugar. Cut each biscuit in half and roll into balls. Dip the balls in butter, then roll in cinnamon sugar. Place 4 balls in each muffin cup. Sprinkle each pull-apart with 1 teaspoon of raisins. Bake for 15–17 minutes, until the biscuits are cooked through.

Serving: 1 pull-apart

210 calories
6 g fat
37 g carbohydrate
3 g protein

Soft Bean Burrito

1 PORTION

½ cup	canned fat-free refried beans
¼ cup	yellow onion, chopped (1.5 ounces)
1 ounce	Mexican-blend cheese, shredded
¼ cup	hot sauce
1	2-ounce flour tortilla

Preheat the oven to 350°F. In a bowl combine the beans, onion, half the cheese, and 2 tablespoons of hot sauce. Place the bean mixture in the center of the tortilla and roll it up. Place the burrito in a small baking dish. Top with the remaining hot sauce and cheese. Bake for 15 minutes, until the burrito is heated through and the cheese is melted.

440 calories
15 g fat
57 g carbohydrate
20 g protein

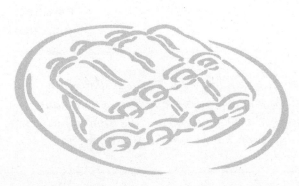

Barbecue Chicken

6 PORTIONS

⅓ cup	ketchup
⅓ cup	tomato juice
2 tablespoons	honey
2 tablespoons	brown sugar, packed
1 teaspoon	dehydrated onion flakes
½ teaspoon	dehydrated minced garlic
¾ teaspoon	black pepper
6	4-ounce boneless, skinless chicken breasts

In a small saucepan combine the ketchup, tomato juice, honey, brown sugar, onion flakes, minced garlic, and black pepper. Bring to a simmer over medium heat and allow to cook at least 15 minutes before using.

Preheat a grill or broiler. Toss the chicken with ½ cup of the barbecue sauce. Grill or broil until cooked through, 6–8 minutes per side, basting with the remaining sauce.

Serving: 1 chicken breast

180 calories
1.5 g fat
15 g carbohydrate
26 g protein

Helpful Tip
This barbecue sauce can be modified with a few changes to be great with pork. Apples and pork are a classic combination, so exchange the honey for maple syrup and the tomato juice for apple. Follow the directions above, substituting pork chops for chicken breasts.

Cheddar and Chive Mashed Potatoes

6 PORTIONS

2 pounds	baking potatoes, peeled and chopped (6 cups)
2 ounces	cheddar cheese, shredded
1 tablespoon	freeze-dried chives
¼ cup	light sour cream
⅓ cup	skim milk
1 teaspoon	kosher salt
⅛ teaspoon	black pepper

Cover the potatoes with cold, salted water. Bring to a boil over high heat and cook until tender, 20–30 minutes. Drain well. Place in the bowl of a stand mixer. Add the cheese, chives, sour cream, milk, salt, and pepper. Whip until smooth.

Serving: ¾ cup

170 calories
4.5 g fat
28 g carbohydrate
3 g protein

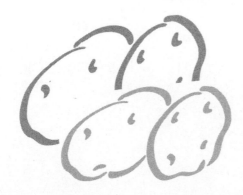

Green Beans with Red Onion and Red Pepper

6 PORTIONS

24 ounces	green beans, washed and trimmed
1 tablespoon	unsalted butter
1½ cups	red onion, sliced thin (6 ounces)
½ teaspoon	kosher salt
⅛ teaspoon	crushed red pepper

Bring a large pot of water to a boil. Cook the green beans for 3–4 minutes, until tender crisp. Drain well, and then rinse immediately with cold water so the beans will not continue to cook.

Melt the butter in a large nonstick skillet over medium-high heat. Add the red onion, salt, and crushed red pepper. Sauté for 5–7 minutes, until the onions become tender. Add the beans to the pan and cook for 1–2 minutes to rewarm the beans and evenly distribute the onion and red pepper flakes.

Serving: ⅔ cup

60 calories
2 g fat
11 g carbohydrate
2 g protein

Day Twenty-One

Breakfast

Banana Muffins	(200 calories)
1 cup skim milk	(90 calories)

Lunch

Chicken, Corn, and Orzo Soup	(210 calories)
Honey Drop Biscuits	(150 calories)
1 medium (6-ounce) pear	(100 calories)

Dinner

Mahimahi with Pineapple Salsa	(180 calories)
Cilantro Couscous	(200 calories)
Buttered Sugar Snap Peas	(60 calories)
1 cup skim milk	(90 calories)

Snacks

320 calories

Banana Muffins

6 PORTIONS

2 tablespoons	unsalted butter, softened
½ cup	granulated sugar
½ cup	liquid egg substitute
½ cup	ripe banana, mashed
1 cup	all-purpose flour
½ teaspoon	baking soda
⅛ teaspoon	iodized salt
½ cup	1% buttermilk

Preheat the oven to 350°F. Cream together the butter and sugar. Stir in the egg substitute and banana and beat until smooth.

Stir together the flour, soda, and salt. Alternate adding the flour mixture and the buttermilk, beginning and ending with the flour. Line a 12-cup muffin pan with paper liners. Divide the batter between the cups, about 3 tablespoons per muffin. Bake for 22–25 minutes, until a tester comes out of the center clean and the top of the muffin springs back if pressed.

Serving: 2 muffins

220 calories
5 g fat
37 g carbohydrate
6 g protein

Helpful Tip
Don't throw overripe bananas away. Pop them in the freezer until the next time you make muffins.

Chicken, Corn, and Orzo Soup

6 PORTIONS

1 tablespoon	unsalted butter
1 cup	yellow onion, chopped (5½ ounces)
1 cup	baby carrots, chopped (5 ounces)
1 cup	celery, chopped (4 ounces)
16 ounces	bone-in, skinless chicken breast
1½ cups	frozen whole kernel corn (9 ounces)
6 cups	fat-free, low-sodium chicken broth
1	bay leaf
1 cup	water
¼ cup	all-purpose flour
½ cup	orzo pasta (4 ounces)
	kosher salt
	black pepper

Melt the butter in a large pot over medium-high heat. Once melted, add the onion, carrots, and celery. Sauté until the vegetables begin to soften, 5–7 minutes. Then add the chicken, corn, broth, and bay leaf to the pot. Bring to a simmer, before turning the heat to medium low. Cook the chicken through, about 30 minutes. Remove the chicken from the pot and set aside to cool.

In a small bowl whisk together the water and flour to produce a smooth paste. Add the flour mixture to the pot along with the orzo. Bring the pot back to a gentle boil and cook 10–15 minutes until the soup thickens and the pasta is cooked.

When the chicken is cool enough to handle, remove the meat from the bones and cut into bite-sized pieces before returning to the soup, discarding the bones. Season with salt and pepper to taste and allow the chicken to rewarm before serving.

Serving: 1½ cups

210 calories
3.5 g fat
32 g carbohydrate
14 g protein

Honey Drop Biscuits

6 PORTIONS

1 cup	all-purpose flour (5 ounces)
1 tablespoon	granulated sugar
¾ teaspoon	baking powder
⅛ teaspoon	baking soda
⅛ teaspoon	iodized salt
	pinch cinnamon
3 tablespoons	unsalted butter, diced, cold
1 tablespoon	honey
3 tablespoons	skim milk

Preheat the oven to 375°F. In a large bowl whisk together the flour, sugar, baking powder, baking soda, salt, and cinnamon. With a pastry blender or two forks, work in the butter until the dry ingredients resemble coarse meal. Stir together the honey and skim milk before adding to the dry ingredients. Mix just until the liquid is incorporated. Drop the dough into six biscuits on a baking sheet and bake 18–20 minutes until lightly browned.

Serving: 1 biscuit

150 calories
6 g fat
21 g carbohydrate
2 g protein

Mahimahi with Pineapple Salsa

6 PORTIONS

6	4-ounce mahimahi fillets
2 tablespoons	olive oil
1	lime
	kosher salt
	black pepper
2	Roma tomatoes, seeded and diced
¾ cup	crushed pineapple, in juice
3 tablespoons	red onion, minced
1 clove	garlic, minced
1 tablespoon	pickled jalapeño peppers, minced
2 tablespoons	cilantro, minced

Preheat the oven to 350°F. Place the mahimahi skin side down on a baking sheet. Brush with olive oil and drizzle with lime juice before seasoning with salt and pepper. Bake the fish for 20–25 minutes, just until it begins to flake.

While the fish is baking, prepare the salsa. Combine the tomatoes, pineapple, red onion, garlic, jalapeños, and cilantro. Allow the salsa to rest for at least 15 minutes before serving.

Serving: 1 mahimahi fillet with ⅓ cup salsa

180 calories
6 g fat
4 g carbohydrate
28 g protein

Cilantro Couscous

6 PORTIONS

3 cups	fat-free, low-sodium chicken broth
1 tablespoon	unsalted butter
½ teaspoon	kosher salt
	pinch black pepper
1½ cups	couscous (9 ounces)
¼ cup	scallions, sliced thin
¼ cup	cilantro, minced

In a large saucepan bring the broth to a boil with the butter, salt, and pepper. Remove from the heat, add the couscous, and cover for 5 minutes. Once the broth is absorbed, remove the lid and fluff the couscous with a fork. Stir in the scallions and cilantro.

Serving: ⅔ cup

200 calories
3 g fat
34 g carbohydrate
8 g protein

Buttered Sugar Snap Peas

6 PORTIONS

24 ounces	sugar snap peas, washed and trimmed
1 tablespoon	unsalted butter
½ teaspoon	kosher salt
	pinch black pepper

Bring a large pot of water to a boil. Boil the peas for 4–5 minutes, until tender. Drain well. Toss with the butter, salt, and pepper.

Serving: ½ cup

60 calories
2.5 g fat
8 g carbohydrate
3 g protein

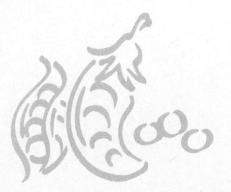

Day Twenty-Two

Breakfast

6 ounces fat-free vanilla yogurt	(90 calories)
1 ounce granola cereal	(105 calories)
½ cup fresh or frozen raspberries	(30 calories)

Lunch

2 1-ounce slices white bread	(160 calories)
2 ounces lean deli roast beef	(80 calories)
¾ ounce cheddar cheese	(80 calories)
1 tablespoon reduced-fat mayonnaise	(25 calories)
1 ounce baked barbecue potato chips	(115 calories)
½ cup unsweetened applesauce	(50 calories)

Dinner

Chili Stuffed Peppers	(220 calories)
Mexican Rice	(180 calories)
Zucchini with Tomatoes and Cumin	(30 calories)
1 cup skim milk	(90 calories)

Snacks

345 calories

Chili Stuffed Peppers

6 PORTIONS

3	large green bell peppers (7 ounces each)
1 pound	96% extra-lean ground beef
1/3 cup	yellow cornmeal (1 1/2 ounces)
1/3 cup	tomato juice
1/4 cup	yellow onion, chopped (1 1/2 ounces)
1	large egg
1/2 teaspoon	chili powder
1/4 teaspoon	ground cumin
1/4 teaspoon	kosher salt
3	3/4-ounce slices cheddar cheese, halved

Chili Sauce

1 16-ounce can	tomato sauce
1 teaspoon	chili power
1/2 teaspoon	ground cumin

Preheat the oven to 350°F. Bring a large pot of water to a boil over high heat. Halve the bell peppers lengthwise and remove the veins and seeds. Boil for 5 minutes, then drain. Place the peppers cut side up in a 9-by-13-inch ovenproof baking pan.

In a large bowl combine the ground beef, cornmeal, tomato juice, onion, egg, chili powder, cumin, and salt. Divide the meat mixture between the six pepper halves, packing the filling into their cavities. Place the peppers in the oven and bake for 20 minutes.

While the peppers are baking, make the chili sauce by combining the tomato sauce, chili powder, and cumin in a small saucepan. Bring to a boil, then simmer for 15 minutes. After the peppers have baked for 20 minutes, top them with the chili sauce and half a slice of cheese. Bake for 10 additional minutes, until the cheese is melted and the peppers are cooked through.

Serving: half of a pepper

220 calories,
8 g fat
18 g carbohydrate
25 g protein

Mexican Rice

6 PORTIONS

1 teaspoon	canola oil
¼ cup	yellow onion, chopped (1½ ounces)
2 cloves	garlic, minced
¼ cup	green bell pepper, chopped (1½ ounces)
1½ cups	basmati rice (9 ounces)
1 tablespoon	canned mild green chilies, chopped
1 teaspoon	chili powder
¼ teaspoon	ground cumin
1 teaspoon	kosher salt
2 cups	low-fat beef broth
1 cup	tomato juice

Heat the oil over medium-high heat in a medium saucepan. Add the onion, garlic, and bell pepper and sauté for 5 minutes, until the onion becomes translucent. Stir in the rice, chilies, chili powder, cumin, and salt. Cook for 1 minute. Add the beef broth and tomato juice and bring to a boil. Turn the heat to low and cover the pan, allowing the rice to simmer 20–25 minutes, until all the liquid is absorbed.

Serving: ⅔ cup

180 calories
1 g fat
37 g carbohydrate
4 g protein

Zucchini with Tomatoes and Cumin

6 PORTIONS

24 ounces	zucchini
1 teaspoon	canola oil
1 clove	garlic, minced
1 teaspoon	whole cumin seed
⅛ teaspoon	crushed red pepper
1 cup	Roma tomato, chopped (6 ounces)
1 teaspoon	kosher salt

Quarter the zucchini and cut into 1-inch chunks. Place the oil, garlic, cumin seed, and crushed red pepper in a cold non-stick skillet. Cook over medium-high heat, until the cumin becomes fragrant and garlic begins to brown lightly, 2–3 minutes. Add the tomatoes, zucchini, and salt. Cover and turn the heat down to medium low. Allow to cook for 5–7 minutes, until the zucchini is tender. Uncover and turn the heat up to high, until any liquid that has collected evaporates.

Serving: ½ cup

30 calories
1 g fat
5 g carbohydrate
2 g protein

Day Twenty-Three

Breakfast

Breakfast Sandwich	(250 calories)
1 medium (3-ounce) plum	(50 calories)

Lunch

Sloppy Joes	(260 calories)
1 ounce Doritos chips	(140 calories)
½ cup mandarin orange segments in juice	(40 calories)

Dinner

Chicken à la King	(370 calories)
Buttered Cauliflower	(45 calories)
1 cup skim milk	(90 calories)

Snacks

310 calories

Breakfast Sandwich

1 PORTION

1	2-ounce plain English muffin
	cooking spray
¼ cup	liquid egg substitute
	kosher salt
	black pepper
1 slice	2% American cheese

Toast the English muffin. Coat a small nonstick skillet with cooking spray. Season the egg substitute with salt and pepper, then scramble over medium heat until cooked through. Mound the eggs in the center of the skillet and top with the cheese. Cook for 2–3 minutes over low heat, until the cheese is melted. Place the egg on half of the English muffin and top with the other half.

250 calories
8 g fat
28 g carbohydrate
17 g protein

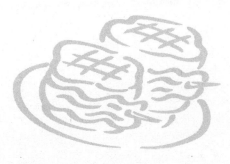

Sloppy Joes

6 PORTIONS

1 pound	96% extra-lean ground beef
2 tablespoons	dehydrated onion flakes
¾ cup	ketchup
1 tablespoon	brown sugar, packed
1 tablespoon	yellow mustard
1 tablespoon	distilled vinegar
6	1½ -ounce hamburger buns

In a large skillet, brown the beef with the onion flakes, stirring frequently to break up the beef. When the beef is cooked through, add the ketchup, brown sugar, mustard, and vinegar. Cook 4–5 more minutes until a thick sauce has formed around the meat. Divide the sloppy joe meat between the 6 hamburger buns.

Serving: ⅓ cup meat, 1 bun

260 calories
4.5 g fat
34 g carbohydrate
23 g protein

Chicken à la King

6 PORTIONS

2 tablespoons	unsalted butter
6	4-ounce boneless, skinless chicken breasts
½ cup	yellow onion, chopped (2½ ounces)
½ cup	canned mushrooms
¼ cup	canned roasted red bell pepper, drained and diced
1 cup	fat-free, low-sodium chicken broth
1 cup	2% milk
3 tablespoons	all-purpose flour
1 teaspoon	kosher salt
¼ teaspoon	black pepper
3 cups	water
1½ cups	basmati rice (9 ounces)

Melt the butter in a large skillet over medium-high heat. Pat the chicken dry and season with the salt and pepper. Brown on both sides, 4–5 minutes per side. Remove the chicken to a plate and add the onion, sautéing for 5 minutes, until tender. Add the mushrooms and bell peppers and cook 5 minutes more.

In a bowl whisk together the chicken broth, milk, flour, salt, and pepper. Turn the pan to medium low and add the milk mixture. Cook the sauce until it thickens, 10–15 minutes, being careful not to break the milk mixture. When the sauce has come to a simmer and thickened, return the chicken to the pan and allow the sauce and chicken to cook 10–15 minutes longer, until the chicken is cooked through.

In a separate saucepan bring the water to a boil with the rice. Once to a boil, cover and turn the heat to low, allowing the rice to cook 20–25 minutes, until all the water is absorbed.

Serving: ¾ cup basmati rice, 1 chicken breast, ½ cup sauce

370 calories
7 g fat
44 g carbohydrate
32 g protein

> *Helpful Tip*
> *What do we mean by "break"? Lower-fat milk products tend to separate if heated too high, leaving behind a curdled mess, otherwise known as breaking.*

Buttered Cauliflower

6 PORTIONS

24 ounces	cauliflower florets
1 tablespoon	unsalted butter, melted
	kosher salt
	black pepper

Place a steamer basket in the bottom of a large pot with a tight-fitting lid. Fill the base of the pot with water, cover, and bring the water to a boil. Once boiling, add the cauliflower, cover, and allow to steam 10–12 minutes, until tender. Remove the cauliflower from the steamer and toss with the butter, salt, and pepper.

Serving: ⅔ cup

45 calories
2 g fat
6 g carbohydrate
2 g protein

Day Twenty-Four

Breakfast

2 low-fat frozen waffles   (235 calories)
2 tablespoons maple syrup   (100 calories)
1 cup honeydew   (60 calories)

Lunch

Asian Chicken Salad with
  Sesame Vinaigrette   (290 calories)
6 sesame crackers   (90 calories)

Dinner

Italian-Seasoned Pork Tenderloin   (160 calories)
Orzo Primavera   (190 calories)
Sugar Snap Pea and Pecorino Salad (90 calories)
1 cup skim milk   (90 calories)

Snacks

295 calories

Asian Chicken Salad

1 PORTION

1	4-ounce boneless, skinless chicken breast
4 ounces	romaine lettuce
2 tablespoons	red onion, diced (½ ounce)
¼ cup	cucumber, peeled and diced
¼ cup	mandarin orange segments in juice
1	serving Sesame Vinaigrette (see recipe that follows)

Grill or broil the chicken breast until cooked through, 6–8 minutes per side. Slice the chicken into thin strips, then toss with the lettuce, red onion, cucumber, and mandarin oranges. Top with Sesame Vinaigrette.

290 calories
15 g fat
12 g carbohydrate
29 g protein

Sesame Vinaigrette

1 PORTION

1 teaspoon	sesame seeds
1 tablespoon	seasoned rice vinegar
2 teaspoons	canola oil
1 teaspoon	toasted sesame oil
1 tablespoon	fresh minced cilantro
1 tablespoon	fresh minced mint
	pinch kosher salt

Over low heat in a small skillet, toast the sesame seeds until golden brown, about 5 minutes. Remove from the heat and allow to cool before using.

In a small bowl whisk together the vinegar and oils. Add the cilantro, mint, sesame seeds, and salt. Allow to rest for at least 15 minutes before using.

120 calories
13 g fat
1 g carbohydrate
0 g protein

Italian-Seasoned Pork Tenderloin

6 PORTIONS

1 teaspoon	kosher salt
1 teaspoon	dried parsley
½ teaspoon	dried basil
½ teaspoon	garlic powder
¼ teaspoon	lemon pepper
⅛ teaspoon	crushed red pepper
⅛ teaspoon	dried oregano
	pinch dried rosemary
2	1-pound pork tenderloins

Preheat the oven to 325°F. In a small bowl combine the salt, parsley, basil, garlic powder, lemon pepper, crushed red pepper, oregano, and rosemary. Pat the pork tenderloins dry and season with the Italian herb seasoning. Allow the pork to marinate for 15 minutes and up to overnight. Roast in the oven for 25–30 minutes, until the tenderloin reaches an internal temperature of 145°F. Remove from the oven, cover with foil, and allow the meat to rest for at least 15 minutes before slicing each tenderloin in thirds.

Serving: ⅓ of a tenderloin

160 calories
4.5 g fat
0 g carbohydrate
31 g protein

Orzo Primavera

6 PORTIONS

1 tablespoon	olive oil
1 cup	canned roasted red bell pepper, drained and diced
1 cup	red onion, chopped (5½ ounces)
1 cup	baby carrots, diced (5 ounces)
3 cloves	garlic, minced
1 cup	orzo pasta (8 ounces)
1 teaspoon	kosher salt
½ teaspoon	dried basil
⅛ teaspoon	dried oregano
⅛ teaspoon	crushed red pepper
2 cups	fat-free, low-sodium chicken broth

Heat the olive oil in a large skillet over medium-high heat. Add the bell pepper, onion, carrots, and garlic and sauté until the onion becomes translucent, 5 minutes. Stir in the orzo and continue to cook until the pasta turns a golden brown. Stir in the salt, basil, oregano, and crushed red pepper, and cook 1 minute more. Add the broth and bring to a boil. Cover and turn the heat down to low. Cook the orzo for 20–25 minutes, until it is tender and the broth is completely absorbed.

Serving: ⅔ cup

190 calories
3 g fat
35 g carbohydrate
6 g protein

Sugar Snap Pea and Pecorino Salad

6 PORTIONS

24 ounces	sugar snap peas, washed and trimmed
1 tablespoon	olive oil
½ tablespoon	red wine vinegar
1 teaspoon	garlic, minced
½ teaspoon	dried oregano
⅛ teaspoon	dried thyme
½ teaspoon	kosher salt
	pinch black pepper
1 ounce	Pecorino cheese, grated

Bring a large pot of water to a boil. Boil the peas for 3–4 minutes, until tender but still crisp. Drain and immediately rinse with cold water so the peas will not continue to cook. Chill. In a large bowl combine the olive oil, red wine vinegar, garlic, oregano, thyme, salt, and pepper. Add the grated Pecorino cheese, then toss the peas with the dressing. Chill for at least 15 minutes more before serving.

Serving: ½ cup

90 calories
4 g fat
8 g carbohydrate
5 g protein

> *Helpful Tip*
> *Can't find Pecorino cheese? Freshly grated Parmesan is a great substitution.*

Day Twenty-Five

Breakfast

1 ounce bran flakes	(100 calories)
½ cup skim milk	(45 calories)
1 medium (5-ounce) banana	(90 calories)

Lunch

Open-Faced Chicken Quesadillas	(475 calories)
Fresh Tomato Salsa	(15 calories)

Dinner

Tuna Noodle Casserole	(440 calories)
⅔ cup prepared frozen peas and carrots	(50 calories)
1 cup skim milk	(90 calories)

Snacks

295 calories

Open-Faced Chicken Quesadillas

1 PORTION

1 teaspoon	canola oil
1	4-ounce boneless, skinless chicken breast
½ cup	yellow onion, chopped (3 ounces)
2 tablespoons	canned mild green chilies
2	1-ounce flour tortillas
1 ounce	Mexican-blend cheese, shredded

Preheat the broiler. Heat the oil in a medium-size nonstick skillet. Finely dice the raw chicken. Sauté the chicken with the onion and green chilies until cooked through, 10–12 minutes. Place the tortillas on a baking sheet and top each with half of the chicken mixture, then half the cheese. Broil for 5–7 minutes, until the cheese is melted and the tortillas are crisp around the edges. Top with Fresh Tomato Salsa (see recipe that follows).

475 calories
19 g fat
36 g carbohydrate
29 g protein

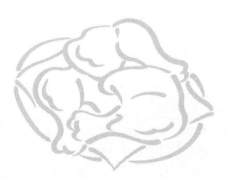

Fresh Tomato Salsa

1 PORTION

1	Roma tomato, seeded and diced
1 tablespoon	red onion, finely diced
1 teaspoon	pickled jalapeño pepper, minced
1 teaspoon	fresh cilantro, minced
1 teaspoon	fresh lime juice
	pinch kosher salt

Combine all the ingredients in a bowl and allow to rest at least 15 minutes before serving.

15 calories
0 g fat
4 g carbohydrate
0 g protein

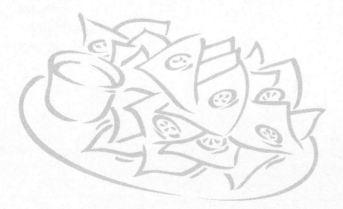

Tuna Noodle Casserole

6 PORTIONS

12 ounces	egg noodles
1 cup	cooking liquid, reserved
2 10¾-ounce cans	cream of mushroom soup
4 ounces	light Velveeta processed cheese
2 6-ounce cans	solid white albacore tuna in spring water

Bring a large pot of salted water to a boil and cook the noodles according to the package directions. Drain the noodles, reserving 1 cup of cooking liquid.

Combine the reserved liquid with the soup and cheese in a large saucepan over medium heat. Once the cheese is melted, add the tuna, including the juice, breaking it up into small chunks. Add the noodles and continue to cook for 5 minutes more, until the mixture is thoroughly combined and heated through.

Serving: 1½ cups

440 calories
15 g fat
50 g carbohydrate
27 g protein

Day Twenty-Six

Breakfast

Cheddar Grits   (210 calories)
1 large (6-ounce) peach   (70 calories)

Lunch

Tuna Salad   (120 calories)
2 1-ounce slices whole wheat bread   (150 calories)
1 ounce baked potato chips   (115 calories)
1 medium (6-ounce) pear   (100 calories)

Dinner

Teriyaki Chicken with Green Beans   (270 calories)
Vegetable Lo Mein   (180 calories)
1 cup skim milk   (90 calories)

Snacks

                                      295 calories

Cheddar Grits

1 PORTION

1	1-ounce packet instant grits
1 ounce	cheddar cheese, shredded
	pinch kosher salt
	pinch black pepper
	pinch garlic powder
	dash hot sauce (optional)

Prepare the grits as the package directs. Stir in the cheese, heating if necessary to fully melt it. Season with salt, pepper, garlic powder, and hot sauce.

210 calories
10 g fat
22 g carbohydrate
9 g protein

Tuna Salad

6 PORTIONS

2 6-ounce cans	solid white albacore tuna in spring water
¼ cup	yellow onion, chopped (1½ ounces)
½ cup	celery, chopped (2 ounces)
1	large egg, hard-boiled and grated
½ cup	reduced-fat mayonnaise
2 tablespoons	sweet pickle, minced
	pinch black pepper

Drain the tuna well, then flake into small pieces before adding the onion, celery, egg, mayonnaise, pickle, and black pepper. Mix until the salad is well combined. Chill or serve immediately.

Serving: ⅓ cup

120 calories
4 g fat
3 g carbohydrate
16 g protein

Teriyaki Chicken with Green Beans

6 PORTIONS

1 cup	low-sodium soy sauce
¼ cup	Japanese rice wine (mirin)
2 cloves	garlic, minced
1 teaspoon	ginger, minced
¼ cup	brown sugar, packed
2 tablespoons	granulated sugar
½ teaspoon	chili-garlic sauce
1½ pounds	boneless, skinless chicken breasts, sliced thin
24 ounces	green beans, washed and trimmed
1 tablespoon	peanut oil
3 tablespoons	cornstarch

In a medium bowl, combine the soy sauce, rice wine, garlic, ginger, sugars, and chili-garlic sauce. Add the chicken and marinate for at least 15 minutes.

Bring a large pot of water to a boil. Add the green beans and boil 3–4 minutes, until tender crisp. Drain the beans well and rinse with cold water to stop them from cooking further.

In a large skillet, heat the oil over medium-high heat. Remove the chicken from the marinade, reserving the marinade, and add it to the skillet. Sauté the chicken until cooked through, stirring frequently. While the chicken cooks, stir the cornstarch into the reserved marinade. Once the chicken is cooked through, add the teriyaki to the pan, and bring to a boil to thicken. Stir in the green beans, tossing with the chicken and sauce to coat.

Serving: 1 generous cup

270 calories
4 g fat
29 g carbohydrate
31 g protein

Vegetable Lo Mein

6 PORTIONS

8 ounces	fresh lo mein noodles
1 tablespoon	peanut oil
1 cup	yellow onion, chopped (5½ ounces)
1 cup	celery, sliced thin (4 ounces)
1 cup	baby carrots, sliced thin (5 ounces)
4 ounces	button mushrooms, sliced
2 cloves	garlic, minced
½ cup	fat-free, low-sodium chicken broth
2 tablespoons	low-sodium soy sauce
1 teaspoon	toasted sesame oil
1 tablespoon	cornstarch
½ cup	bean sprouts, cleaned
¼ cup	scallions, sliced thin

Bring a large pot of water to a boil. Prepare the noodles according to the package directions. In a large skillet, heat the peanut oil until almost smoking. Add the onion, celery, carrots, mushrooms, and garlic and sauté until they just begin to soften. In a small bowl combine the chicken broth, soy sauce, sesame oil, and cornstarch. Add to the pan and bring to a boil and thicken. Add the drained noodles, stirring to evenly coat with sauce. Stir in the bean sprouts and scallions before serving.

Serving: 1 cup

180 calories
4 g fat
30 g carbohydrate
6 g protein

Day Twenty-Seven

Breakfast

Brown Sugar Apple Butter Muffins	(240 calories)
1 cup skim milk	(90 calories)

Lunch

Chicken Vegetable Soup	(250 calories)
1 1-ounce slice whole wheat bread	(75 calories)
¾ ounce cheddar cheese	(80 calories)
1 cup sweet cherries	(85 calories)

Dinner

Braised Pork with Rosemary and Thyme	(180 calories)
Mushroom Pilaf	(160 calories)
Buttered Carrots	(50 calories)
1 cup skim milk	(90 calories)

Snacks

340 calories

Brown Sugar Apple Butter Muffins

6 PORTIONS

2 tablespoons	unsalted butter, softened
½ cup	brown sugar, packed
½ cup	liquid egg substitute
½ cup	apple butter
1 cup	all-purpose flour
½ teaspoon	baking soda
½ teaspoon	ground cinnamon
¼ teaspoon	ground nutmeg
⅛ teaspoon	iodized salt
½ cup	1% buttermilk

Preheat the oven to 350°F. Cream together the butter and brown sugar. Stir in the egg substitute and apple butter and beat until smooth.

Stir together the flour, baking soda, cinnamon, nutmeg, and salt. Alternate adding the flour mixture and buttermilk, beginning and ending with the flour. Line a 12-cup muffin pan with paper liners. Divide the batter between the cups, about 3 tablespoons per muffin. Bake for 22–25 minutes, until a tester comes out of the center clean and the top of the muffin springs back if pressed.

Serving: 2 muffins

240 calories
4.5 g fat
44 g carbohydrate
5 g protein

Chicken Vegetable Soup

6 PORTIONS

12 ounces	boneless, skinless chicken breast, diced
1½ cups	yellow onion, chopped (8 ounces)
1 cup	celery, chopped (4 ounces)
1 cup	baby carrots, chopped (5 ounces)
1 cup	frozen green beans (4½ ounces)
1 cup	frozen baby lima beans (6 ounces)
1 cup	frozen peas (5 ounces)
1 cup	frozen whole kernel corn (6 ounces)
1 28-ounce can	petite diced tomatoes
4 cups	fat-free, low-sodium chicken broth
1	bay leaf
½ teaspoon	dried thyme
¼ teaspoon	black pepper

Combine all the ingredients in a large pot. Bring to a simmer over medium heat. Allow to simmer 2–3 hours before serving.

Serving: 1½ cups

250 calories
2.5 g fat
35 g carbohydrate
23 g protein

Braised Pork with Rosemary and Thyme

6 PORTIONS

1	2-pound center-cut pork loin
	kosher salt
	black pepper
1 head	garlic, halved
1 sprig	fresh rosemary
1 sprig	fresh thyme
2	bay leaves

Preheat the oven to 300°F. Season the pork loin with salt and pepper, then place in a 4-quart casserole dish with a tight-fitting lid. Surround the pork with the garlic, rosemary, thyme, and bay leaves. Add 2–3 cups of water, enough to cover the pork. Place the lid on the casserole before placing the pork in the oven. Braise for 2–3 hours, until the pork is fork tender. Remove the pork from the oven and uncover, allowing it to rest 15–20 minutes before serving.

180 calories
4.5 g fat
4 g carbohydrate
31 g protein

Helpful Tip
This recipe works wonderfully in a Crock-Pot. Place the pork and seasoning in large Crock-Pot and fill with water. Cook the pork loin on the lower setting for 6–8 hours.

Mushroom Pilaf

6 PORTIONS

2 tablespoons	unsalted butter
½ cup	yellow onion, chopped (3 ounces)
1 cup	basmati rice (6 ounces)
1 cup	canned mushrooms, drained
2 cups	low-fat, low-sodium beef broth
1 teaspoon	Worcestershire sauce
1 teaspoon	kosher salt
¼ teaspoon	black pepper

Melt the butter in a large skillet over medium heat. Add the onions and cook until tender, about 5 minutes. Stir in the rice, cooking until it begins to brown, 2–3 minutes. Add the mushrooms, beef broth, Worcestershire sauce, salt, and pepper. Bring the broth to a boil, then cover and turn to low. Allow the rice to cook 20–25 minutes, until all the liquid is absorbed.

Serving: ¾ cup

160 calories
4 g fat
27 g carbohydrate
4 g protein

Buttered Carrots

6 PORTIONS

1 14-ounce can	fat-free, low-sodium chicken broth
1 tablespoon	unsalted butter
1 pound	baby carrots
	kosher salt
	black pepper

In a large skillet bring the broth and butter to a boil. Add the carrots and continue to boil until the broth has evaporated, 15–20 minutes. The carrots should be tender and coated with the broth and butter reduction. Season to taste with salt and pepper.

Serving: ½ cup

50 calories
2.5 g fat
7 g carbohydrate
1 g protein

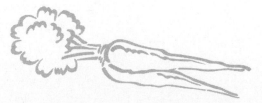

Day Twenty-Eight

Breakfast

2 large eggs, scrambled	(140 calories)
1 1-ounce slice whole wheat bread	(75 calories)
³/₄ ounce cheddar cheese	(80 calories)
1 cup skim milk	(90 calories)

Lunch

Tarragon Chicken Salad	(220 calories)
1 2-ounce French roll	(140 calories)
Marinated Asparagus	(70 calories)

Dinner

Mustard and Cheese Cod	(200 calories)
Parsley and Buttered New Potatoes	(140 calories)
Roasted Sea Asparagus	(40 calories)
1 cup skim milk	(90 calories)

Snacks

315 calories

Tarragon Chicken Salad

6 PORTIONS

1½ pounds	boneless, skinless chicken breast
1	Granny Smith apple, peeled and diced (5-ounce)
1 ounce	walnut pieces, toasted
¾ cup	celery, diced (3 ounces)
2 tablespoons	scallions, sliced thin
½ cup	reduced-fat mayonnaise
¼ cup	light sour cream
2 teaspoons	fresh tarragon, minced
¾ teaspoon	kosher salt
	pinch black pepper

Place the chicken in a large saucepan and cover with cold water. Bring to a boil over high heat, turn heat to low, and simmer for 15–20 minutes, until cooked through. Cool to room temperature, then cut or pull into bite-sized pieces.

Combine the chicken, apple, walnuts, celery, and scallions in a large bowl. In a medium bowl stir together the mayonnaise, sour cream, tarragon, salt, and pepper. Toss the tarragon dressing with the chicken mixture. The salad may be chilled several hours or served immediately.

Serving: ⅔ cup

220 calories
9 g fat
6 g carbohydrate
28 g protein

Helpful Tip
Can't find fresh herbs? Trade ⅓ of the fresh amount for dried.
For this recipe, substitute ¾ teaspoon dried tarragon.

Marinated Asparagus

6 PORTIONS

24 ounces	asparagus spears
2 tablespoons	olive oil
1 tablespoon	tarragon vinegar*
	kosher salt
	black pepper

*A good-quality white vinegar may be substituted for the tarragon vinegar.

Bring a large pot of water to a boil. Wash the asparagus and trim the woody ends (last 2–3 inches) from the spears. Boil for 2 minutes, drain, and rinse under cold water. Pat dry.

Whisk together the oil and vinegar. Toss with the asparagus and season with salt and pepper. Refrigerate for at least 15 minutes before serving.

Serving: 3 ounces

70 calories
4.5 g fat
5 g carbohydrate
3 g protein

Mustard and Cheese Cod

6 PORTIONS

6	*4-ounce cod fillets*
1½ cups	*2% milk*
3 tablespoons	*all-purpose flour*
3 ounces	*cheddar cheese, shredded*
1 teaspoon	*dry mustard*
	kosher salt
	black pepper

Preheat the oven to 350°F. In a small saucepan, whisk together the milk, flour, cheese, and mustard. Bring to a simmer over medium heat, until thickened and smooth, 10–15 minutes.

While the sauce is cooking, place the cod fillets in a 9-by-13-inch baking dish. Season with salt and pepper. Once the sauce is thickened, pour it over the fish. Place the cod in the oven and bake for 20–25 minutes, until it just begins to flake.

Serving: 1 fillet and ⅓ cup sauce

200 calories
7 g fat
6 g carbohydrate
26 g protein

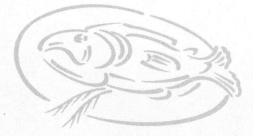

Parsley and Buttered New Potatoes

6 PORTIONS

2 pounds	*small red potatoes*
2 tablespoons	*unsalted butter*
¼ cup	*fresh parsley, minced*
1 teaspoon	*kosher salt*
¼ teaspoon	*black pepper*

Leave the potatoes whole, or halve, depending on their size. Place in a large pot and cover with cold, salted water. Bring to a boil and cook until fork tender, 30–40 minutes, depending on the size of the potatoes. Drain well and toss with the butter, parsley, salt, and pepper.

Serving: ¾ cup

140 calories
4 g fat
27 g carbohydrate
0 g protein

Roasted Sea Asparagus

6 PORTIONS

24 ounces	*sea asparagus*
	cooking spray
	kosher salt
	black pepper

Preheat the oven to 400°F. Wash the sea asparagus and trim the stems and discard. Arrange in a single layer on a foil-lined baking sheet. Coat the sea asparagus evenly with cooking spray. Roast 5–7 minutes, depending on the thickness of the spears. Remove from the oven and season with salt and pepper.

Serving: 3 ounces

40 calories
.5 g fat
8 g carbohydrate
1 g protein

Helpful Tip
Sea asparagus—also known as samphire—is similar in shape to traditional asparagus with ends reminiscent of broccoli. Seasonably available in the summer months, it is a great substitute for asparagus or any other vegetable that is roasted.

Snack Guide

Fruit

Apple, medium (5½-ounce)	90	calories
Apples, dried (1 ounce)	75	calories
Applesauce, sweetened (½ cup)	90	calories
Applesauce, unsweetened (½ cup)	50	calories
Apricots, dried (1 ounce)	65	calories
Banana, medium (4-ounce)	80	calories
Blueberries/blackberries (½ cup)	40	calories
Cantaloupe (1 cup)	60	calories
Cherries, sweet (1 cup)	85	calories
Cranberries, sweetened, dried (1 ounce)	95	calories
Currants, dried (1 ounce)	80	calories
Fig pieces, dried (1 ounce)	70	calories
Fruit gelatin, sugar-free (½ cup)	10	calories
Fruit gelatin, sugared (½ cup)	85	calories
Fruit gelatin with fruit (½ cup)	80	calories
Fruit sherbet/sorbet (½ cup)	120	calories
Grapefruit, ½ (10 ounces)	55	calories
Grapes, red or green (1 cup)	100	calories
Honeydew (1 cup)	60	calories
Kiwifruit, medium (3-ounce)	45	calories
Mandarin orange segments in juice (½ cup)	40	calories
Nectarine, medium (4-ounce)	50	calories
Orange, medium (7-ounce)	70	calories
Peach, medium (4-ounce)	35	calories
Peaches, canned in juice (½ cup)	55	calories
Pear, medium (6-ounce)	90	calories
Pears, canned in juice (½ cup)	60	calories
Pineapple (1 cup)	75	calories
Pineapple chunks canned in juice (½ cup)	70	calories
Pineapple tidbits, dried (1 ounce)	80	calories

Plum, medium (3-ounce)	45	calories
Prunes with pits (1 ounce)	60	calories
Raisins (1 ounce)	90	calories
Raspberries (½ cup)	30	calories
Strawberries (1 cup)	45	calories
Tangerine, medium (4-ounce)	50	calories
Watermelon (1 cup)	50	calories

Nuts

Almonds (1 ounce)	170	calories
Cashews (1 ounce)	165	calories
Mixed nuts (1 ounce)	175	calories
Peanut butter (1 tablespoon)	105	calories
Peanuts (1 ounce)	165	calories
Pecans (1 ounce)	190	calories
Sunflower seed kernels (1 ounce)	160	calories
Walnuts (1 ounce)	175	calories

Dairy

Cheddar cheese (¾ ounce)	80	calories
Cojack cheese (¾ ounce)	80	calories
Cottage cheese, low-fat (½ cup)	80	calories
Fudge bar, nonfat	60	calories
Orange Creamsicle	110	calories
Pudding, nonfat chocolate/vanilla (½ cup)	100	calories
String cheese (1 ounce)	80	calories
Swiss cheese (¾ ounce)	80	calories
Yogurt, nonfat, fruit (6 ounces)	90	calories
Yogurt, low-fat, frozen (½ cup)	120	calories
Yogurt, nonfat, frozen (½ cup)	100	calories

Chips/Cookies/Crackers

Animal crackers (1 ounce)	120	calories
Chips Ahoy! chocolate chip cookies (3 cookies)	160	calories
Club crackers (4 crackers)	70	calories
Doritos chips (1 ounce)	140	calories
Fig Newtons (2 cookies)	220	calories
Ginger snaps (5 cookies)	150	calories
Goldfish snacks (1 ounce)	140	calories
Graham crackers (8 crackers)	120	calories
Nutty Bars (2 ounces)	155	calories
Popcorn, 94% fat-free (1 cup)	25	calories
Potato chips, baked (1 ounce)	110	calories

Pretzels, fat-free (1 ounce)	110	calories
Oatmeal Creme Pie	170	calories
Oreo cookies (3 cookies)	160	calories
Ritz Chips (1 ounce)	135	calories
Triscuit crackers (1 ounce)	130	calories
Vanilla wafers (10 cookies)	150	calories
Vienna Fingers (2 cookies)	140	calories
Wheat Thins (1 ounce)	135	calories

Beverage Guide

Aside from specifying milk in the daily plans, we have left beverage selection up to you. Obviously, if you make caloric choices, those calories must come from your snack allowance. Sugar-free drinks such as water, tea, coffee, and of course, diet Dr Pepper, are free.

Juice/Lemonade

Apple juice (6 fluid ounces)	90	calories
Cranberry juice (6 fluid ounces)	100	calories
Fruit punch (6 fluid ounces)	85	calories
Grape juice (6 fluid ounces)	125	calories
Grapefruit juice (6 fluid ounces)	70	calories
Lemonade (12 fluid ounces)	170	calories
Lemonade, diet (12 fluid ounces)	25	calories
Orange juice (6 fluid ounces)	80	calories
Tomato juice (6 fluid ounces)	30	calories
V8 juice (12 fluid ounces)	70	calories

Milk (8 fluid ounces)

Milk, skim	90	calories
Milk, 1%	125	calories
Milk, 2%	140	calories
Milk, chocolate, 2%	190	calories
Milk, whole	150	calories

Soda Products (12 ounces)

Coca-Cola Classic	160	calories
Coca-Cola Classic, caffeine-free	145	calories

Diet Coke	0	calories
Cherry Coke	155	calories
Vanilla Coke	150	calories
Dr Pepper	150	calories
Diet Dr Pepper	0	calories
Mountain Dew	185	calories
Mountain Dew, caffeine-free	185	calories
Diet Mountain Dew	0	calories
Pepsi	165	calories
Diet Pepsi	0	calories
Pepsi Vanilla	170	calories
Wild Cherry Pepsi	160	calories
7-Up	150	calories
Diet 7-Up	0	calories
Sprite	145	calories
Diet Sprite	0	calories

Coffee/Tea

Coffee, decaffeinated (6 fluid ounces)	0	calories
Coffee, regular (6 fluid ounces)	5	calories
Iced tea, sweetened (12 fluid ounces)	150	calories
Iced tea, unsweetened (12 fluid ounces)	5	calories
Tea, regular, no milk or sugar (8 fluid ounces)	0	calories
Tea, herbal (8 fluid ounces)	5	calories

Alcohol

Beer, regular (16 fluid ounces)	200	calories
Beer, light (16 fluid ounces)	135	calories
Wine cooler (12 fluid ounces)	210	calories
Wine, red (4 fluid ounces)	85	calories
Wine, white, dry (4 fluid ounces)	80	calories
Wine, white, sweet (4 fluid ounces)	85	calories
Liqueurs (1 fluid ounce)		
Amaretto	110	calories
Baileys Irish Cream	95	calories
Chambord	105	calories
Cointreau	100	calories
Crème de cacao	100	calories
Crème de menthe	120	calories
Drambuie	105	calories
Frangelico	80	calories
Galliano	100	calories
Grand Marnier	100	calories
Kahlúa	100	calories
Kirsch	80	calories

Midori	80	calories
Ouzo	90	calories
Pernod	75	calories
Sambuca	100	calories
Schnapps	100	calories
Tia Maria	90	calories
Triple Sec	80	calories

Liquors (1 fluid ounce)*

Brandy	70	calories
Cognac	70	calories
Gin	80	calories
Rum	70	calories
Tequila	65	calories
Vodka	70	calories
Whiskey, bourbon	70	calories
Whiskey, scotch	70	calories

*Calories based on 80 proof alcohol

Jamba Juice—all calories based on Original-sized beverages

JUICES

Carrot	160	calories
Lemonade	455	calories
Orange/Banana	370	calories
Orange/Carrot	260	calories
Orange	340	calories
Vibrant-C	395	calories

SMOOTHIES

Aloha Pineapple	515	calories
Banana Berry	475	calories
Berry Lime Sublime	455	calories
Caribbean Passion	440	calories
Chocolate Moo'd	730	calories
Citrus Squeeze	480	calories
Coldbuster!	445	calories
Cranberry Craze	445	calories
Enlightened, Berry Fulfilling	295	calories
Enlightened, Mango Mantra	335	calories
Enlightened, Strawberry Nirvana	300	calories
Jamba Powerboost	455	calories
Kiwi Berry Burner	470	calories
Mango-A-Go-Go	440	calories

Orange-A-Peel	455	calories
Orange Berry Blitz	420	calories
Orange Dream Machine	540	calories
Peach Pleasure	465	calories
Peanut Butter Moo'd	885	calories
Peenya Kowlada	690	calories
Protein Berry Pizzazz	460	calories
Razzmatazz	480	calories
Strawberries Wild	450	calories

Starbucks—all calories based on grande-sized beverages, and where applicable made with whole milk

COFFEE

Caffè Americano	15	calories
Caffè Latte	260	calories
Café au Lait	140	calories
Caffè Mocha, no whipped cream	300	calories
Caffè Mocha, with whipped cream	400	calories
Cappuccino	150	calories
Caramel Macchiato	310	calories
Caramel Mocha, no whipped cream	370	calories
Caramel Mocha, with whipped cream	470	calories
Coffee of the Week, no milk or sugar	10	calories
Decaf Coffee of the Week, no milk or sugar	10	calories
Syrup-Flavored Latte	280	calories
Toffee Nut Crème, no whipped cream	350	calories
Toffee Nut Crème, with whipped cream	460	calories
Vanilla Crème, no whipped cream	330	calories
Vanilla Crème, with whipped cream	440	calories

FRAPPUCCINO BLENDED COFFEE

Caffè Vanilla, no whipped cream	340	calories
Caffè Vanilla, with whipped cream	470	calories
Caffè Vanilla, light, no whipped cream	230	calories
Caffè Vanilla, light, with whipped cream	360	calories
Caramel, no whipped cream	280	calories
Caramel, with whipped cream	430	calories
Caramel, light, no whipped cream	180	calories

Caramel, light, with whipped cream	310	calories
Caramel Mocha, no whipped cream	330	calories
Caramel Mocha, with whipped cream	460	calories
Caramel Mocha, light, no whipped cream	230	calories
Caramel Mocha, light, with whipped cream	360	calories
Coffee	260	calories
Coffee, light, no whipped cream	150	calories
Coffee, light, with whipped cream	280	calories
Espresso	230	calories
Espresso, light, no whipped cream	140	calories
Espresso, light, with whipped cream	270	calories
Java Chip, no whipped cream	370	calories
Java Chip, with whipped cream	510	calories
Java Chip, light, no whipped cream	260	calories
Java Chip, light, with whipped cream	400	calories
Mocha, no whipped cream	290	calories
Mocha, with whipped cream	420	calories
Mocha, light, no whipped cream	180	calories
Mocha, light, with whipped cream	310	calories
Toffee Nut, no whipped cream	280	calories
Toffee Nut, with whipped cream	420	calories
White Chocolate Mocha, no whipped cream	320	calories
White Chocolate Mocha, with whipped cream	450	calories
White Chocolate Mocha, light, no whipped cream	200	calories
White Chocolate Mocha, light, with whipped cream	340	calories

ICED COFFEE

Caffè Americano	20	calories
Caffè Latte	160	calories
Caffè Mocha, no whipped cream	220	calories
Caffè Mocha, with whipped cream	350	calories
Caramel Macchiato	270	calories
Caramel Mocha, no whipped cream	290	calories
Caramel Mocha, with whipped cream	420	calories
Shaken Coffee	80	calories
Syrup-Flavored Latte	210	calories
Vanilla Latte	210	calories

White Chocolate Mocha, no whipped cream	360	calories
White Chocolate Mocha, with whipped cream	490	calories

NON-COFFEE BEVERAGES

Apple juice	230	calories
Chocolate Milk	340	calories
Hot Chocolate, no whipped cream	340	calories
Hot Chocolate, with whipped cream	440	calories
White Hot Chocolate, no whipped cream	480	calories
White Hot Chocolate, with whipped cream	580	calories

TAZO TEA

Iced Tazo Chai Tea Latte	270	calories
Tazo Chai Tea Latte	290	calories
Tazo Iced Tea	80	calories
Tazo Tea Lemonade	120	calories

Fast-Food Guide

ATLANTA BREAD COMPANY

Bagels

Asiago Cheese	380	calories
Apple Spice	360	calories
Blueberry	270	calories
Cinnamon Crisp	330	calories
Everything	320	calories
Onion	290	calories
Plain	270	calories
Poppy Seed	320	calories
Sesame	360	calories
Wheat	270	calories

Cream Cheese (2 ounces)

Garden Vegetable	170	calories
Onion & Chive	190	calories
Plain	190	calories
Plain, light	120	calories
Strawberry	190	calories

Breads

French roll	160	calories
Sourdough roll	160	calories

Sandwiches

ABC Special on French, no mayo or cheese	420	calories
Hot Pastrami, no mayo or cheese	460	calories
Tangy Roast Beef, no horseradish, cheddar, or mayo	390	calories

Cup of Soup

Black Bean with Ham	250	calories
Chicken Tortilla	190	calories
Chunky Baked Potato	290	calories
Classic Chicken Noodle	140	calories
Cream of Broccoli	200	calories
Cream of Tomato	130	calories
French Onion	80	calories
French Onion with toppings	200	calories
Frontier Chicken Chili	270	calories
Garden Vegetable	100	calories
Hearty Beef Chili	350	calories
Homestyle Chicken and Dumplings	290	calories
New England Clam Chowder	280	calories
Pasta Fagioli	170	calories
Spicy Chicken Gumbo	120	calories
Wisconsin Cheese	240	calories

BACK YARD BURGERS

Sandwiches/Entrees

Back Yard Burger Jr.	310	calories
Back Yard Hot Dog	310	calories
Back Yard BLT	270	calories
Blackened Chicken Sandwich	290	calories
Garden Veggie Sandwich	240	calories
Savory Chicken Sandwich	230	calories

Hawaiian Chicken Sandwich	280	calories
Honey Mustard Chicken Sandwich	320	calories
Lemon Butter Chicken Sandwich	260	calories
Barbecue Chicken Sandwich	280	calories
Bacon Swiss Chicken Sandwich	390	calories

Chicken Strips and Nuggets

Chicken Tenderloins (3 pieces)	400	calories

Sauces

Gravy Dipping Sauce	70	calories
Barbecue Dipping Sauce	50	calories

Salads

Garden Salad	25	calories
Asian Chicken Salad	460	calories
Blackened Chicken Salad	160	calories
Charbroiled Chicken Salad	140	calories
Chicken Club Salad	430	calories

Salad Dressing

Ranch dressing (1 packet)	270	calories
Italian dressing (1 packet)	200	calories
Honey Mustard dressing (1 packet)	140	calories
Thousand Island dressing (1 packet)	250	calories
Fat-Free Ranch dressing (1 packet)	60	calories
Fat-Free Italian dressing (1 packet)	20	calories
Fat-Free Honey Dijon dressing (1 packet)	60	calories

Sides

Cup of Chili	270	calories
Traditional Baked Potato	170	calories
Chili and Cheddar Baked Potato	330	calories
Ranch Baked Potato	410	calories
Salsa Baked Potato	250	calories
Seasoned Fries, regular	260	calories
Waffle Fries, regular	240	calories

BLIMPIE

Cold Subs—6-inch subs on white with cheese (except Seafood & Tuna), lettuce, tomato, and onion

Blimpie Best	476	calories
Club	440	calories
Ham & Cheese	436	calories

Roast Beef	468	calories
Seafood	355	calories
Tuna	493	calories
Turkey	424	calories

Hot Subs—6-inch subs on white with cheese (except Grilled Chicken, MexiMax, and VegiMax), lettuce, tomato, and onion

Grilled Chicken	373	calories
Buffalo Chicken	400	calories
Steak & Onion Melt	440	calories
MexiMax	425	calories
VegiMax	395	calories

Salads

Antipasto	244	calories
Chef	212	calories
Grilled Chicken (with Caesar dressing)	347	calories
Seafood	122	calories
Tuna	261	calories
Zesto Pesto Turkey	370	calories
Roast Beef 'n Bleu	390	calories

Sides

Cole Slaw	180	calories
Mustard Potato Salad	160	calories
Potato Salad	270	calories

Soups

Chicken Soup with White & Wild Rice	230	calories
Tomato Basil with Raviolini	110	calories
Grande Chili with Beans & Beef	250	calories
Vegetable Beef	80	calories
Cream of Potato	190	calories
Homestyle Chicken Noodle	120	calories
Cream of Broccoli & Cheese	190	calories
Garden Vegetable	80	calories

BURGER KING

Breakfast

Croissan'wich with Bacon, Egg & Cheese	340	calories
Croissan'wich with Ham, Egg & Cheese	340	calories

Croissan'wich with Sausage
  & Cheese   410   calories
Croissan'wich with Egg & Cheese   300   calories
French Toast Sticks   390   calories
Hash Brown Rounds, small   230   calories
Grape Jam (½ ounce)   30   calories
Strawberry Jam (½ ounce)   30   calories
Breakfast Syrup (1 ounce)   80   calories

Sandwiches
  Original Whopper Jr.   390   calories
  Original Whopper Jr., no
    mayonnaise   310   calories
  Original Whopper Jr., with
    cheese   430   calories
  Original Whopper Jr., with cheese,
    no mayonnaise   350   calories
  Hamburger   310   calories
  Cheeseburger   350   calories
  BK Veggie Burger   380   calories
  BK Veggie Burger, no mayonnaise   300   calories
  Chicken Whopper, no mayonnaise   410   calories
  Chicken Whopper Jr., no
    mayonnaise   320   calories
  BK Big Fish Sandwich, without
    tartar sauce   360   calories

Chicken Strips and Nuggets
  Chicken Tenders (4 pieces)   170   calories
  Chicken Tenders (5 pieces)   210   calories
  Chicken Tenders (6 pieces)   250   calories
  Chicken Tenders (8 pieces)   340   calories

Sauces
  Barbecue Dipping Sauce   35   calories
  Honey Flavored Dipping Sauce   90   calories
  Honey Mustard Dipping Sauce   90   calories
  Sweet and Sour Dipping Sauce   40   calories
  Ranch Dipping Sauce   140   calories
  Zesty Onion Ring Dipping Sauce   150   calories
  Ketchup (1 packet)   10   calories

Salads
  Side Garden Salad   20   calories
  Fire-Grilled Chicken Caesar Salad   190   calories
  Fire-Grilled Shrimp Caesar Salad   180   calories

Tendercrisp Caesar Salad	390	calories
Fire-Grilled Chicken Garden Salad	210	calories
Fire-Grilled Shrimp Garden Salad	200	calories
Tendercrisp Garden Salad	410	calories

Salad Dressings and Toppings

Garden Ranch (2 ounces)	120	calories
Creamy Garlic Caesar (2 ounces)	130	calories
Sweet Onion Vinaigrette (2 ounces)	100	calories
Tomato Balsamic Vinaigrette (2 ounces)	110	calories
Fat-Free Honey Mustard Dressing (2 ounces)	70	calories
Garlic Parmesan Toast	70	calories

Sides

Small Fries	230	calories
Small Onion Rings	180	calories

CHICK-FIL-A

Breakfast

Biscuit	260	calories
Chick-n-Minis, 3-count	270	calories
Chick-n-Minis, 4-count	360	calories
Chicken Biscuit	420	calories
Bacon, Egg & Cheese Biscuit	470	calories
Sausage Biscuit	490	calories
Biscuit and Gravy	330	calories
Chicken Breakfast Burrito	420	calories
Sausage Breakfast Burrito	460	calories
Bagel, no butter or cream cheese	220	calories
Chicken, Egg & Cheese Bagel	460	calories
Hashbrowns	260	calories

Sandwiches

Chicken Sandwich	410	calories
Chicken Sandwich, no butter	380	calories
Chicken Deluxe Sandwich	420	calories
Chargrilled Chicken Sandwich	270	calories
Chargrilled Chicken Club Sandwich	380	calories
Chicken Salad Sandwich	350	calories
Spicy Chicken Cool Wrap	380	calories
Chargrilled Chicken Cool Wrap	390	calories
Chicken Caesar Cool Wrap	460	calories

Chicken Strips and Nuggets
Chick-n-Strips (4-count)	290	calories
Chick-n-Strips (6-count)	430	calories
Nuggets (4-pack)	130	calories
Nuggets (6-pack)	200	calories
Nuggets (8-pack)	260	calories
Nuggets (12-pack)	290	calories

Sauces
Polynesian Sauce (1 ounce)	110	calories
Barbecue Sauce (1 ounce)	45	calories
Honey Mustard Sauce (1 ounce)	45	calories
Buttermilk Ranch Sauce (¾ ounce)	110	calories
Buffalo Sauce (¾ ounce)	15	calories
Honey Roasted BBQ Sauce (.4 ounce)	60	calories

Salads
Chargrilled Chicken Garden Salad	180	calories
Chick-n-Strips Salad	390	calories
Southwest Chargrilled Salad	240	calories

Salad Dressings and Toppings
Caesar Dressing (1 packet)	400	calories
Reduced Fat Raspberry Vinaigrette (1 packet)	160	calories
Buttermilk Ranch Dressing (1 packet)	400	calories
Blue Cheese Dressing (1 packet)	375	calories
Spicy Dressing (1 packet)	350	calories
Thousand Island Dressing (1 packet)	375	calories
Light Italian Dressing (1 packet)	30	calories
Fat-Free Honey Mustard (1 packet)	120	calories
Garlic and Butter Croutons	50	calories
Honey Roasted Sunflower Kernels	80	calories
Tortilla Strips	70	calories

Sides
Waffle Potato Fries, small	270	calories
Fresh Fruit Cup	60	calories
Carrot & Raisin Salad	170	calories
Cole Slaw	180	calories
Side Salad	60	calories
Hearty Breast of Chicken Soup, regular	140	calories
Hearty Breast of Chicken Soup, large	250	calories
Chicken Salad Cup	270	calories

FAZOLI'S

Sandwiches

Grilled Chicken Panini	420	calories

Pasta

Spaghetti with Marinara Sauce, small	440	calories
Spaghetti with Meat Sauce, small	460	calories
Fettuccine Alfredo, small	490	calories
Classic Ziti with Meat Sauce, small	430	calories
Penne Marinara	430	calories

Salads

Garden Side Salad, no dressing	25	calories
Caesar Side Salad, no dressing	110	calories
Chicken Caesar Salad, no dressing	190	calories
Pasta Side Salad, no dressing	240	calories
Chicken and Pasta Caesar Salad	360	calories
Grilled Chicken Salad	110	calories

Soups

Minestrone Soup	90	calories
Herbed Chicken Noodle Soup	70	calories
Tomato Florentine Soup	130	calories
Three Meatballs	260	calories

Sides

Breadstick	140	calories
Breadstick, no butter	100	calories

Desserts

Lemon Italian Ice	190	calories

MCDONALD'S

Breakfast

Egg McMuffin	290	calories
Sausage McMuffin	370	calories
English Muffin	150	calories
Biscuit	240	calories
Sausage Burrito	300	calories
Sausage Patty	170	calories
Scrambled Eggs (2)	180	calories
Hash Browns	140	calories

Grape Jam (1 packet)	35	calories
Strawberry Preserves (1 packet)	35	calories

Sandwiches

Hamburger	260	calories
Cheeseburger	310	calories
Double Cheeseburger	460	calories
Quarter Pounder	420	calories
Quarter Pounder with Cheese	510	calories
Filet-O-Fish	400	calories
Chicken McGrill	400	calories
Crispy Chicken	500	calories
McChicken	420	calories
Hot 'n Spicy McChicken	440	calories

Chicken Nuggets and Strips

Chicken McNuggets (4-piece)	170	calories
Chicken McNuggets (6-piece)	250	calories
Chicken McNuggets (10-piece)	420	calories
Chicken Selects (3-piece)	380	calories

Sauces

Ketchup (1 packet)	10	calories
Barbecue Sauce (1 packet)	45	calories
Honey (1 packet)	50	calories
Hot Mustard Sauce (1 packet)	50	calories
Sweet 'N Sour Sauce (1 packet)	50	calories
Spicy Buffalo Sauce (1 packet)	60	calories
Creamy Ranch Sauce (1 packet)	200	calories
Tangy Honey Mustard Sauce (1 packet)	70	calories
Chipotle Barbecue Sauce (1 packet)	70	calories

Salads

Bacon Ranch Salad	130	calories
Bacon Ranch Salad with Grilled Chicken	240	calories
Bacon Ranch Salad with Crispy Chicken	340	calories
Caesar Salad	90	calories
Caesar Salad with Grilled Chicken	200	calories
Caesar Salad with Crispy Chicken	300	calories
California Cobb Salad	150	calories

California Cobb Salad with Grilled Chicken	260	calories
California Cobb Salad with Crispy Chicken	360	calories
Side Salad	15	calories

Salad Dressings and Toppings

Newman's Own Cobb Dressing	120	calories
Newman's Own Creamy Caesar Dressing	190	calories
Newman's Own Low-Fat Balsamic Vinaigrette	40	calories
Newman's Own Ranch Dressing	170	calories
Butter Garlic Croutons	60	calories

Sides

French Fries, small	230	calories
French Fries, medium	350	calories

Desserts

Fruit 'n Yogurt Parfait	160	calories
Fruit 'n Yogurt Parfait, no granola	130	calories
Apple Dippers with Low Fat Caramel Dip	100	calories
Apple Dippers	35	calories
Vanilla Reduced Fat Ice Cream Cone	150	calories
Kiddie Cone	45	calories
Strawberry Sundae	280	calories
Hot Caramel Sundae	340	calories
Hot Fudge Sundae	330	calories
Peanuts for sundaes	45	calories
Baked Apple Pie	250	calories
McDonaldland Chocolate Chip Cookies	270	calories
McDonaldland Cookies	250	calories

PANERA BREAD

Bagels

Asiago Cheese Bagel	330	calories
Blueberry Bagel	320	calories
Chocolate Raspberry Bagel	370	calories
Cinnamon Crunch Bagel	420	calories
Dutch Apple & Raisin Bagel	340	calories

Everything Bagel	290	calories
French Toast Bagel	340	calories
Nine Grain Bagel	290	calories
Plain Bagel	280	calories
Pumpkin Spice Bagel	360	calories
Sesame Bagel	310	calories

Spreads (2 ounces)

Plain Cream Cheese	190	calories
Reduced Fat Hazelnut Cream Cheese	150	calories
Reduced Fat Honey Walnut Cream Cheese	150	calories
Reduced Fat Mocha Cream Cheese	160	calories
Reduced Fat Plain Cream Cheese	130	calories
Reduced Fat Raspberry Cream Cheese	120	calories
Reduced Fat Sun-Dried Tomato Cream Cheese	140	calories
Reduced Fat Veggie Cream Cheese	130	calories

Breads

French Roll	140	calories
Sourdough Roll	160	calories

Sandwiches

Asiago Roast Beef	730	calories
Bacon Turkey Bravo	770	calories
Chicken Salad on Nine Grain	640	calories
Coronado Carnitas Panini	810	calories
Frontega Chicken Panini	860	calories
Garden Veggie	570	calories
Peanut Butter & Jelly on French	450	calories
Pepperblue Steak Sandwich	780	calories
Pesto Roma Club	650	calories
Portobello & Mozzarella Panini	670	calories
Sierra Turkey	950	calories
Smoked Ham & Swiss on Rye	650	calories
Smoked Turkey Breast on Sourdough	440	calories
Smokehouse Turkey Panini on Asiago Focaccia	840	calories
Tuna Salad on Honey Wheat	720	calories
Turkey Artichoke Panini	810	calories
Tuscan Chicken	950	calories

Soups

Asparagus & Chicken Florentine Soup	230	calories
Baked Potato Soup	260	calories
Boston Clam Chowder	210	calories
Broccoli Cheddar Soup	230	calories
Cream of Chicken & Wild Rice Soup	200	calories
French Onion Soup with cheese & croutons	220	calories
Low-Fat Chicken Noodle Soup	100	calories
Low-Fat Vegetarian Autumn Tomato Basil Soup	110	calories
Low-Fat Vegetarian Black Bean Soup	160	calories
Low-Fat Vegetarian Garden Vegetable Soup	90	calories

Salads

Asian Sesame Chicken Salad	330	calories
Bistro Steak Salad	630	calories
Caesar Salad	390	calories
Classic Café Salad	390	calories
Fandango Salad	400	calories
Grilled Chicken Caesar Salad	500	calories
Greek Salad	520	calories
Tomato & Fresh Mozzarella Salad	790	calories

SUBWAY

Cold Sandwiches—6-inch sandwiches on Italian or wheat bread with lettuce, tomatoes, onions, green peppers, pickles, and olives

Honey Mustard Chicken	320	calories
Oven Roasted Chicken Breast	330	calories
Roast Beef	290	calories
Savory Turkey Breast	280	calories
Savory Turkey Breast & Ham	290	calories
Subway Club	320	calories
Sweet Onion and Chicken Teriyaki	370	calories
Veggie Delite	230	calories
Classic Tuna with cheese	530	calories
Cold Cut Combo with cheese	410	calories
Subway Seafood Sensation with cheese	450	calories

Hot Sandwiches—6-inch sandwiches on Italian or wheat bread with lettuce, tomatoes, onions, green peppers, pickles, olives, and cheese

Cheese Steak	360	calories
Chicken & Bacon Ranch	530	calories
Chipotle Southwest Cheese Steak	450	calories
Italian BMT	450	calories
Meatball Marinara	560	calories
Turkey Breast, Ham & Bacon Melt	380	calories

Deli-Style Sandwiches—Deli roll with lettuce, tomatoes, onions, green peppers, pickles, and olives

Classic Tuna	350	calories
Ham	210	calories
Roast Beef	220	calories
Savory Turkey Breast	210	calories

Wraps

Chicken & Bacon Ranch with cheese	440	calories
Tuna with cheese	440	calories
Turkey Breast & Bacon Melt with Chipotle Sauce	440	calories
Turkey Breast	190	calories

Salads (dressing and croutons not included)

Grilled Chicken & Baby Spinach	140	calories
Subway Club	160	calories
Tuna with cheese	360	calories
Veggie Delite	60	calories

Salad Dressings

Honey Mustard (2 ounces)	200	calories
Greek Vinaigrette (2 ounces)	200	calories
Fat-Free Italian (2 ounces)	35	calories
Ranch (2 ounces)	200	calories

WENDY'S

Sandwiches

Jr. Hamburger	280	calories
Jr. Cheeseburger	320	calories
Jr. Cheeseburger Deluxe	360	calories
Jr. Bacon Cheeseburger	380	calories
Classic Single with Everything	430	calories
Ultimate Chicken Grill Sandwich	360	calories

Spicy Chicken Fillet Sandwich	510	calories
Homestyle Chicken Fillet Sandwich	540	calories

Chicken Strips and Nuggets

Homestyle Chicken Strips (3-piece)	410	calories
Nuggets (4-piece)	180	calories
Nuggets (5-piece)	220	calories

Sauces

Deli Honey Mustard Sauce (1 packet)	170	calories
Spicy Southwest Chipotle Sauce (1 packet)	140	calories
Heartland Ranch Sauce (1 packet)	200	calories
Barbecue Sauce (1 packet)	40	calories
Sweet and Sour Sauce (1 packet)	45	calories
Honey Mustard Sauce (1 packet)	130	calories

Salads

Mandarin Chicken Salad	170	calories
Spring Mix Salad	180	calories
Chicken BLT Salad	330	calories
Taco Supremo Salad	380	calories
Homestyle Chicken Strips Salad	440	calories
Caesar Side Salad	70	calories
Side Salad	35	calories

Salad Dressings and Toppings

Oriental Sesame Dressing (1 packet)	190	calories
House Vinaigrette Dressing (1 packet)	190	calories
Honey Mustard Dressing (1 packet)	280	calories
Homestyle Garlic Croutons (1 packet)	70	calories
Caesar Dressing (1 packet)	150	calories
Fat Free French Style Dressing (1 packet)	80	calories
Reduced Fat Creamy Ranch (1 packet)	100	calories
Low Fat Honey Mustard Dressing (1 packet)	110	calories
Creamy Ranch Dressing (1 packet)	230	calories
Salsa (1 packet)	30	calories
Sour Cream (1 packet)	60	calories
Taco Chips (1 bag)	210	calories
Crispy Noodles (1 packet)	60	calories
Roasted Almonds (1 packet)	130	calories
Honey Roasted Pecans (1 packet)	130	calories

Baked Potatoes

Plain	270	calories
Sour Cream and Chives	340	calories
Broccoli and Cheese	440	calories
Bacon and Cheese	560	calories
Country Crock Spread (1 packet)	60	calories

Chili

Small	220	calories
Large	330	calories
Hot Chili Seasoning (1 packet)	5	calories
Saltine Crackers (1 packet)	25	calories

Sides

Kids' Meal Fries	280	calories

Desserts

Fresh Fruit Bowl	130	calories
Low-Fat Strawberry Flavored Yogurt	90	calories
Mandarin Orange Cup	80	calories
Fresh Fruit Cup	60	calories
Junior Frosty (6-ounce)	160	calories
Small Frosty (12-ounce)	330	calories

Recipe Index

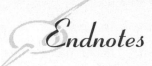
Endnotes

Introduction

1. K. M. Flegal, M. D. Carroll, C. L. Ogden, and C. L. Johnson, "Prevalence and Trends in Obesity among US Adults, 1999–2000." *Journel of the American Medical Association* 288 (2002):1723–27.
2. "Childhood Obesity—Advancing Effective Prevention and Treatment: An Overview for Health Professionals." Issue paper prepared for the National Institute for Health Care Management Research and Educational Foundation Forum, April 9, 2003.

Chapter 1

3. C. L. Ogden, C. D. Fryar, M. D. Carroll, and K. M. Flegal, "Mean Body Weight, Height, and Body Mass Index, United States 1960–2002." Advance data from vital and health statistics; no 347. Hyattsville, MD: National Center for Health Statistics, 2004.
4. SizeUSA National Sizing Survey. The objective of the SizeUSA National Sizing Survey is to measure the body dimensions of a representative sample of the U.S. population using the 3D body scanning technology developed at [TC].
5. 2004 survey completed by Booth Research Services, Inc., for the Calorie Control Council, a nonprofit international association of manufacturers of low-calorie, reduced-fat food and light foods and beverages. www.caloriecontrol.org/pr072704.html
6. M. R. Freedman, J. King, and E. Kennedy, "Popular Diets: A Scientific Review." *Journal of Obesity Research* 9, Suppl. 1 (2001): 33S–34S.
7. G. D. Foster, T. A. Wadden, R. A. Vogt, and G. Brewer, "What Is a Reasonable Weight Loss? Patients' Expectations and Evaluations of Obesity Treatment Outcomes." *Journal of Consulting and Clinical Psychology* 65, no. 1 (1997): 79–85.

Chapter 2

8. National Center for Health Statistics, *Health, United States, 2004. With Chartbook on Trends in the Health of Americans.* Hyattsville, MD: 2004.
9. Northwestern Nutrition. www.feinberg.northwestern.edu/nutrition/factsheets/fad-diets.html

Chapter 3

10. National Institute of Diabetes and Digestive and Kidney Diseases, Weight-control Information Network. www.win.niddk.nih.gov/statistics/index.htm
11. J. L. Groff and S. S. Gropper, *Advanced Nutrition and Human Metabolism,* 3rd ed. Belmont, CA: Wadsworth, 1999.

Chapter 8

12. Economic Research Service, USDA Center for Nutrition Policy and Promotion. December 21, 2004. www.ers.usda.gov/
13. G. Block, "Foods Contributing to Energy Intake in the US: Data from NHANES III and NHANES 1999–2000." *Journal of Food Composition and Analysis* 17, nos. 3–4 (2004): 429–47.
14. B. J. Rolls, "The Role of Energy Density in the Overconsumption of Fat." *Journal of Nutrition* 130 (2000): 268S–271S.

Chapter 9

15. M. Nestle and M. F. Jacobson, "Halting the Obesity Epidemic: A Public Health Policy Approach." *Public Health Reports* 115, no 1 (2000): 12–24.
16. B. J. Rolls, L. S. Roe, J. S. Meengs, and D. E. Wall, "Increasing the Portion Size of a Sandwich Increases Energy Intake." *Journal of the American Dietetic Association* 104, no. 3 (2004): 367–72.

Chapter 10

17. Economic Research Service, USDA Center for Nutrition Policy and Promotion. www.ers.usda.gov/briefing/DietAndHealth/data/nutrients/table5.htm
18. B. H. Lin, J. Guthrie, and J. R. Blaylock, "The Diets of America's Children: Influence of Dining Out, Household Characteristics, and Nutrition Knowledge." Agriculture Economics Report No. (AER746), 48 pp, December 1996.

Chapter 11

19. R. F. Kushner, *Roadmaps for Clinical Practice: Case Studies in Disease Prevention and Health Promotion—Assessment and Management of Adult Obesity: A Primer for Physicians.* Chicago: American Medical Association, 2003.

Chapter 12

20. U.S. Department of Health and Human Services, *Physical Activity and Health: A Report of the Surgeon General.* Atlanta: U.S. Department of Health and Human Services, Centers for Disease Control and Prevention, National Center for Chronic Disease Prevention and Health Promotion, 1996.

Chapter 13

21. Institute of Medicine of the National Academies, *Preventing Childhood Obesity: Health in Balance.* Washington, DC: National Academy of Sciences, 2005.

Chapter 14

22. *Esquire,* February 1994.
23. *Roadmaps for Clinical Practice.*

Chapter 15

24. National Restaurant Association, *Meal Consumption Behavior.* 2000. www.restaurant.org/dineout/nutritionqa.cfm
25. Y. Ma, E. R. Bertone, E. J. Stanek, G. W. Reed, J. R. Hebert, N. L. Cohen, P. A. Merriam, and I. S. Ickene, "Association between eating patterns and obesity in a free-living US adult population." *American Journal of Epidemiology* 158 (2003): 85–92.